Canine Epilepsy

An Owner's Guide to Living With and Without Seizures

Caroline D. Levin RN

Foreword by Lauren K. Chattigré DVM

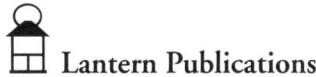

Copyright © May 2002, Caroline D. Levin. All rights reserved. This book may not be reproduced in whole or in part in any manner.

Illustrations and photographs by Caroline Levin (except where otherwise noted).

Cover photograph: "Booker" (Great Dane) trained and posed by Shannon Wilkinson.

First Printing, May 2002
Printed in Canada

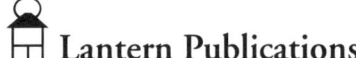 Lantern Publications
18709 S. Grasle Road
Oregon City, OR 97045-8899

www.petcarebooks.com
503-631-3491

ISBN 0-9672253-3-7

LCCN 2002092068

Disclaimer: While every precaution has been taken in providing accurate and relevant information, the material in this book is published for educational purposes only. The author and publisher are not engaged in providing veterinary advice. The reader accepts the information herein with the understanding that healthcare is an individual matter, and that people act on it at their own risk and with full knowledge that veterinary professionals should be consulted for veterinary care.

This book is sold without warranty of any kind, either express or implied. The author, photography models, and publisher assume no responsibility for the care and handling of the reader's dog(s). Neither is any liability assumed from damages resulting from the use of this information or suggestions contained herein.

Dedication

This book is dedicated to Sandra Dobbs and her epileptic dogs "Judy" and "Mitzi" (in spirit). Sandra recognized the need for a guide to canine epilepsy and encouraged me to write it. Without her, this book would not exist. Thank you, Sandra.

Acknowledgements

I would like to extend my sincere thanks to Lauren Chattigré DVM and Albert James Simpson DVM, for their time, knowledge, and support of my work. I have learned much from both of them.

Many thanks to the canine nutritionists who have shared their expertise with me: Darleen Rudnick; Jennifer Boniface, MS; Lisa Newman, PhD; and especially Lew Olson, PhD. Their willingness to teach helped make this book a reality.

I am grateful for all I have learned from Dawn Jecs, my obedience instructor. She possesses a truly brilliant understanding of canine behavior and I am lucky to know her.

I would like to thank my willing and patient photography models: Timothy Shellans; Shannon Wilkinson, certified TTouch practitioner, with her Great Dane, "Booker;" and Natalie Shellans and her English Mastiff, "Columbo." Thanks to Marion Mitchell for providing photographs of her lovely Dalmation, "Emma," and Joeanne Butler for photographing her talented Miniature Schnauzer, "Liza."

Thanks, too, to the dog owners who have shared their experiences, insight, and expertise: Sandra Dobbs, Joanne Carson, Janet Wilson, Heidi Schmeck, Jackie Wyandt, Marion Mitchell, Beth Lagimoniere, Dianne Sever, Linda Jansma, Johanna Thompson, Janice Adams, Phyllis Bsharah, Melinda Miller, Susan McLaughlin, Nancy Cummings, Olivia Bravo, Catherine Dominguez, Christine Reese, Sandie Snider, and Karri Anne Cross.

There are many other dog owners who have answered my questions over the years — too many to name, but all of them important and appreciated.

I thank my family and friends who continually support me as I plow through these projects. As always, I am grateful to my husband, Daniel, without whom my books would not be possible, and to my editor, Andrea Rotondo Hospidor, for all her hard work.

Contents

Preface i
About the Author iii
Foreword v

Chapter 1
Dealing With Loss 1
    Denial 2
    Anger 2
    Bargaining 3
    Depression 3
    Acceptance 4
    Children and Loss 5

Chapter 2
The Doctor-Client Relationship 7
    The Veterinarian's Part 7
    The Dog Owner's Part 8
    Treatment Philosophies 8

Chapter 3
Normal Canine Structure and Function 11
    The Gastrointestinal (GI) Tract 11
    The Endocrine and Immune Systems 13
    Normal Canine Digestion and Metabolism 14
        Carbohydrates 15
        Proteins 16
        Fats (Lipids) 17
        Some Other Important Nutrients 18
    The Brain 20
        Neurons 22
        Cell Membranes 22
        Receptors 23
        Channels 23
        Normal Nerve Transmission 24

Chapter 4
Epilepsy: Definitions and Diagnosis 27
    Defining Epilepsy 27
        Idiopathic/Genetic Causes 28
        Developmental Causes 28
        Nutritional/Metabolic Causes 29
        Additional Causes: Trauma, Tumors, Strokes, Hypoxia, and More 30
    Generalized Seizures 31
    Partial Seizures or Focal Seizures 31
    Cluster Seizures 32
    Status Epilepticus 32
    Diagnosing Epilepsy 33
        Laboratory tests 33
        Electroencephalogram (EEG) 34
        Computerized Axial Tomography (CAT) Scan 34
        Magnetic Resonance Imaging (MRI) 34
        Spinal Tap 34

Chapter 5
Seizure-provoking Factors 37
    Part I: Diet 37
    Commercial Diets 37
        The Benefits of Feeding Commercial Pet Foods 38
        The Drawbacks of Feeding Commercial Pet Foods 38
            Cooking at High Temperatures 40
            Enzymes 41
            Bioavailability and Altered Nutrients 42
            Slowed Digestion 44
            Fiber in Commercial Foods 44
            Fats in Commercial Foods 45
            Chemicals in Commercial Foods 46
            Grains and the Endocrine Pancreas 48
    Part II: Immune System & Endocrine (hormone) Function 50
    A Review of the Immune System 50
    Cortisol — The Stress Hormone 52
        Patterns of Cortisol Release 56
        The High Cortisol Continuum 57
    Part III: Genetics 59
        Cortisol's Relationship to Autoimmune Disease 60
        Thyroid Function, Metabolism, and Seizures 61

Part IV: Additional Environmental Factors 63
    Chemicals, Pesticides, and Wormers 63
    Vaccines 64
    Additional Environmental Triggers 65
Part V: Summary 66

Chapter 6
Overview of Treatments 71
Antiepileptic Drugs (AEDs) 71
Dietary 71
 Environmental 72
Alternative Therapies 72
Surgery 72
Seizure-Arresting Techniques 73
Keeping Notes 73

Chapter 7
Antiepileptic Drugs 75
Phenobarbital (Pb) 76
    Action 76
    Phenobarbital Dosages 76
    Side Effects of Phenobarbital 78
Potassium Bromide (KBr) 78
    Action 78
    Potassium Bromide Dosages 79
    Side Effects of Potassium Bromide 80
Diazepam (or Valium) 80
    Forms of Diazapam/Valium 81
    Action 81
    Diazapam/Valium Dosages 82
    Home Valium Procedure For Cluster Seizures 82
    Preparing a Valium Syringe 83
    Administering Rectal Valium 84
    Side Effects (Valium) 86
Felbamate (or Felbatol) 86
Clonazepam (or Klonopin, Rivotril) 87
Primidone (or Mysoline) 87
Medications Used in Status Epilepticus 87
Medication Refills 87

Chapter 8
Dietary Therapy 89
   A Review of Commercial Diets 89
   More Wholesome Options for Feeding 90
   Diets Prepared at Home 90
      Preparing a Home-cooked Diet 91
         Feeding Dogs With Kidney Disease or Pancreatitis 91
         The Benefits of Feeding Home-cooked Diets 96
         The Drawbacks of Feeding Home-cooked Diets 96
      Raw Food Diets 97
         Preparing a Raw Food Diet 99
         The Benefits of Feeding Raw Food Diets 101
         The Drawbacks of Feeding Raw Food Diets 101
   Variations in Homemade Diets 102
   Switching Diets 102
   Snacks, Treats, and How to Hide Medications 104
   Water Consumption 106
   Changes in Body Weight 106
   Dietary Supplements 107
      Vitamins, Minerals, and Antioxidants 107
      Trace minerals 107
      Amino Acids 108
      Essential Fatty Acids (EFAs) 109
      S-adenosylmethionine (SAMe) 109
      Milk Thistle (Silymarin) 110
      Glandular Extracts 110
      Melatonin 110
      Phosphatidyl Serine (or Phosphatidylserine) 111
      Digestive Enzymes 111

Chapter 9
Alternative Therapies 115
   Acupuncture 115
   Massage 116
   Tellington-Touch 116
   Herbs 118
   Flower Essence Therapy 118
   Physical Exercise 119
   Chiropractic Treatment 119

Chapter 10
Seizures: Before, During, and After 121
- The Seizure Kit 121
- The Phases of a Seizure 122
  - Preictal Phase 122
    - Seizure Alert Dogs 123
    - Arresting Behaviors 125
  - Ictal Phase 127
    - What To Do During a Seizure 127
    - Pack Members' Behaviors 128
  - Postictal Phase 129
    - What To Do After a Seizure 129
    - Document the Seizure Activity in Your Journal: 131
- Bring Your Dog to the Veterinary Clinic When 131

Chapter 11
Additional Health Concerns 133
- Preventive Health Measures 133
  - Physical Assessment 133
  - Other Preventive Measures 134
- Infections 134
  - Skin Infections 135
  - Ear Infections 135
  - Urinary Tract Infections (UTIs) 136
  - Dietary Management of Infection 137
- Renal (Kidney) Problems 137
  - Kidney Infection 137
  - Kidney Degeneration 138
- Incontinence 138
  - Steroid-induced Incontinence 138
  - Treating Incontinence 139
  - Behavioral Issues and Incontinence 139
  - Cleaning Up Accidents 139
  - Dietary Issues and Incontinence 140
  - Mechanical Aids and Items for Incontinence 140
- Hepatic (Liver) Disease 141
- Hypothyroidism: Diagnoses and Treatment 143
  - Thyroid Testing 143
    - AEDs, Cortisol, and Thyroid Tests 144
    - Hypothyroid Treatment 144

Ophthalmic Issues 146
    Blindness Due to Transient Ischemia 147
    Blindness: Sudden Acquired Retinal Degeneration Syndrome (SARD) 147
    Dry Eye Syndrome (keratoconjunctivitis sicca or KCS) 148
    Uveitis 149
    Glaucoma 149
Psychological Stress 150
    Making a Safe Spot 150
    Pack Issues 151
    Separation Anxiety 152
    Changes in Pack Dynamics 153
    Traveling 154
    Competitive Sports and the Epileptic 154
Other Factors That Contribute to Canine Disease 155
    Heartworm Prevention 155
    Flea Control 156
        New Vaccine Protocols 157
Surgical Considerations 158
Epilepsy and Breeding Practices 158
Comfort Measures 159
    Heat Intolerance 159
    Muscle Weakness 160

Chapter 12
Closing Thoughts **163**
Emotional Support 163
A Word About Dog Training 163
The Future 163

Suppliers and Resources 165

Glossary 171

Bibliography 177

Index 185

Other Books by the Author 192

Preface

In the spring of 2001, I finished writing *Dogs, Diet, and Disease*. I had fully intended to spend the coming summer relaxing, tending my garden, and training my puppy. So it came as some surprise when I received a reader's letter proposing an idea for a new book. The reader, Sandra Dobbs, kindly complimented my previous work and then asked me to consider writing about canine epilepsy.

I really hadn't planned to do any further writing for a while but Sandra made a strong case for such a book. She pointed out that many dog owners and veterinarians notice links between thyroid disease, diet, and seizures. She explained with a wink, "So you've already started the research." I agreed.

It wasn't long before I realized a vast and intricate connection between diet, endocrine function, and brain activity. These concepts are gaining serious attention in the field of human healthcare. So much so, that entirely new specialties, such as neuroimmunology and neuroendocrinology, are developing around these connections.

You will learn many helpful things from this book. Some might make you slap your forehead and cry, "Of course! Those are exactly the symptoms my dog has!" Others things may surprise you greatly, so much so, that you may not want to believe them. With this book, you can help your dog have a better quality of life and spare your future pets a lifetime of chronic disease and disorders. Share what you learn with your breeder, your veterinarians, and friends.

In the dog fancy, male dogs are usually referred to as exactly that: "dogs." Females are referred to as "bitches." For ease in writing this book, I've chosen to refer to all canines, both male and female, as "dogs" or "he." This does not represent a higher incidence of illness among males. (I have also referred to all owners as "he.")

Caroline D. Levin RN

About the Author

With a unique combination of personal and professional experiences, Caroline Levin has created another important resource book for dog owners. *Canine Epilepsy* examines one of the most common neurological problems diagnosed in dogs today.

Levin's experience in healthcare began as a registered nurse. She specialized in such fields as ophthalmology, family practice nursing, and endocrinology. After a decade of nursing, Levin left this field to manage an ophthalmic veterinary clinic. It was here that she realized the desperate need blind-dog owners had for educational material. Since then, she has written the first two works on this topic: *Living With Blind Dogs* and *Blind Dog Stories*.

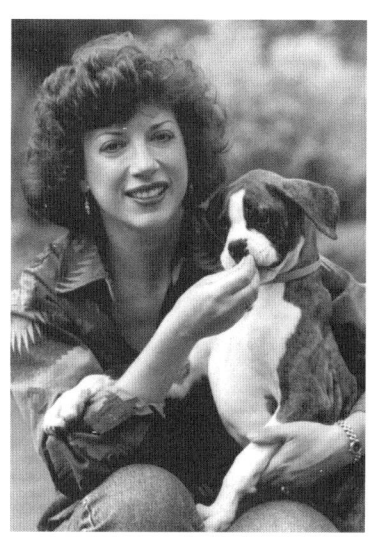

Photo courtesy of Vern Witake

Periodically, Levin's readers contacted her with questions about canine diabetes and its related problems. She realized that there was a need for educational material on these topics, too. Levin scrutinized the current literature, drew on her own nursing background, and consulted with dozens of experts. What began as a small diabetes text, evolved into a dissertation on immune disorders, metabolic disease, endocrine problems, and canine nutrition. The result was her third book, *Dogs, Diet and Disease*, winner of the prestigious Maxwell Award for "Best Healthcare Book 2001."

At the conclusion of that project, Levin was approached by yet another reader who explained the need *epileptic*-dog owners had for educational material. Levin responded to the request by writing *Canine Epilepsy*.

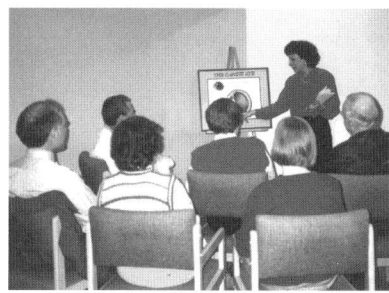

Caroline Levin is also an award-winning dog trainer. She has an in-depth understanding of canine behavior and the methods used to successfully train dogs. She shows her dogs in AKC obedience trials and the new sport of musical canine freestyle. Levin is frequently requested as a guest speaker and has written for a variety of publications.

Foreword

In Traditional Chinese Medicine (TCM), the internal organs are divided into yin and yang pairs. The yin organs are solid (e.g. kidneys); their functions are to produce, transform, regulate, and store. The yang organs are hollow (e.g. bladder); their functions are to receive, break down, absorb, transport, and excrete. The brain, however, falls into a third category called the Curious Organs. They resemble yang in form but yin in function and were given a special place in Chinese medical thinking. Several thousand years later, the brain seems just as curious. Its intricate web of interconnections and close relation with all other body systems — especially the endocrine and immune systems — is something modern medicine has only begun to understand.

This book offers a taste of the interconnections among the neurologicical, endocrine, and immune systems as they relate to brain function and health, particularly with regard to canine epilepsy. Options for medical treatment of epilepsy, both conventional and alternative, are discussed with equal regard. But this book does something else the ancient Chinese would have understood quite well; it highlights the importance of proper diet and stress reduction.

TCM has two main categories of precipitating factors in illness: External (heat, cold, damp, and other environmental influences) and internal (emotional disharmony). However, like the brain, diet and lifestyle have their own category called Way of Life that is considered neither internal nor external. This includes diet, exercise, sexual activity, and occupation. The physician who could intercept imbalance at this level, as well as in the mental/emotional sphere, was considered far superior to the physician who waited until illness was physically manifest because of susceptibility to external influences.

Improper diet is detrimental for obvious reasons: The body is deprived of essential nutrients for basic functioning. But its effects on the immune system, especially in the developing animal, have far-reaching implications for the remainder of the animal's life, and in all other aspects of its physiology. A disharmonious lifestyle, particularly one that is stressful, impacts most directly the endocrine system and cortisol balance in the body. This, too, affects all organs including the brain.

When we think of a stressful lifestyle, we tend to think of people who overwork and have little time for family, and pets can certainly bear the brunt of these stresses. But in a dog's life, we must also consider sources of stress that may not immediately occur to us. For example, the border collie who spends too much time idle, unable to express his natural highly active and inquisitive tendencies, is also experiencing stress. Chinese medicine understands that a harmonious lifestyle cannot be defined as a particular ratio of activities, but rather as a unique way of life that allows one to fully realize and express one's true self.

Diet and lifestyle begin in the home. There is no medicine powerful enough to perfectly compensate for imbalances in these areas. And there is no medicine that could not benefit in its effectiveness from a harmonious Way of Life. People with pets who are ill so often describe feeling powerless to help. How empowering to know then that there are very elemental and important ways in which we can help.

Lauren K. Chattigré DVM, DVetHom, CVA, CVCP, Reiki Master
April 21, 2002

Dr. Chattigré practices holistic veterinary medicine (including acupuncture, Chinese and Western herbology, chiropractic, homeopathy, reiki, and conventional medicine) in Beaverton, Oregon. She also gives public lectures throughout the greater Portland area.

Chapter 1

Dealing With Loss

Many people feel a great sense of loss when their dog is diagnosed with epilepsy. Some may feel overwhelmed after simply skimming through the pages of this book. Others may cry, feel anger, or isolation in their grief. Some owners may even consider euthanizing an epileptic pet. All of these reactions are normal.

There is a particular feeling of helplessness associated with canine epilepsy. It can be frightening to stand by and witness a full-blown seizure. And, it can be worrisome to anticipate the arrival of the next one. As one owner explains it, "There is a distinct type of grief we experience when someone we love goes from being 'whole' to being handicapped."

Some owners are sad for their dog's sake, wondering what quality of life they can expect for their pet. Others are sad for their own sake. They may ask themselves questions such as:

"Will I still love my dog as much as I did before the disease?"
"Will he be as good as everyone else's dog?"
"Will my friends and family pity my dog?"
"Will I be able to provide the necessary care?"
"Will my dog have a happy life or will he be miserable?"

Author Elisabeth Kubler-Ross is well known for her work in the area of grief management. She has outlined five stages people typically experience as they cope with loss: Denial, anger, bargaining, depression, and finally, acceptance. This progression can certainly be applied to the dog owner as he adjusts to his dog's new condition.

Grieving is like a roller-coaster ride with many ups and downs. People experience these stages in varying sequences. Some move through one stage, only to return to it at a later time. Other people may even employ more than one coping mechanism at the same time.

The way in which an individual copes may depend on the nature of the relationship he has with the dog. Someone closely bonded may naturally experience a tremendous amount of grief. Other recent losses in a person's life can compound the intensity of the feeling.

Denial

Initially, a common way to cope with loss is through denial. Denial protects the mind from the bad news being received. A dog owner may seek out a second or third medical opinion, in hopes of hearing that the problem was misdiagnosed or that the dog will experience a miraculous recovery.

When a dog owner is in denial, the situation may seem unreal to him. He may continue daily activities just as if the dog were not ill, even to the point of withholding medical care. During this phase, an owner may distance himself emotionally from his pet. By reducing contact with the dog, the owner can avoid facing his own pain.

Anger

Eventually, denial gives way to anger. This is a time when a dog owner may say to himself, "This is so unfair. Why did this happen to my dog?!"

In normal instances, humans are the caretakers, guardians, and rule-makers for their dogs. In the face of a seizure or sudden illness, a dog owner may feel that he is no longer in control of the situation. This may contribute to his level of anger. An inability to ensure a pet's well-being can be enormously frustrating and even frightening.

It is not uncommon for the dog owner to have angry feelings toward the veterinary staff, as well. In the dog-owner's mind, not only did the veterinarian make this diagnosis, but he is also unable to cure the problem!

Anger may also be expressed toward friends and family members, frequently taking the form of criticism in how they care for the dog. It is important to recognize that such outbursts may only be expressions of the dog-owner's grief.

It is even possible for the owner to express anger toward the dog. He doesn't truly blame the dog for somehow "catching" an illness. He is simply frustrated and wishes he could restore the dog's previous level of health. Happily, dogs are immensely forgiving creatures and may never remember this stage.

Feelings of guilt can be associated with the anger stage. The owner may question his own care of the dog and wonder if something he did could have caused his dog's disease. Such guilt may manifest itself in a number of unhealthy ways. One example is excessive coddling of the dog.

Bargaining

The anger stage is sometimes followed by a bargaining stage. An owner may believe at some level that if denial and anger did not resolve this problem, he may be able to negotiate or bargain for a cure.

The bargaining is usually done secretly, with a Higher Power. One example might be: "If you make my dog well, I will never raise my voice to him again!" Bargaining is a way to keep hope alive. This phase is often short-lived and the dog owner may progress to a state of depression.

Depression

Depression, or sorrow, may set in when the signs of illness can no longer be denied or when seizure activity increases. Some owners mistakenly believe that epilepsy may be a death sentence or, at least, a major disability for their dog. They believe that their most enjoyable activities — such as hiking in the woods or running together on the beach — will be lost.

While friends might try to cheer the grieving pet owner, it is important to allow the transition through this stage. It's essential for each dog owner to give himself permission to grieve. Sorrow is actually a healing emotion. It allows an individual to prepare for the future and accept the realities of caring for an epileptic dog.

The time it takes for a person to move through this stage can vary greatly. There is no predetermined timetable. Eventually the feelings of sadness and helplessness will give way to feelings of acceptance: The final stage.

Acceptance

Acceptance is reached when an individual has had time to work through all the previous stages. There is no average time for this process. As one dog owner puts it, "It takes as long as it takes." Talking with sympathetic friends and enjoying the smallest of pleasures with your dog may help.

Once a dog owner is no longer isolated or in denial, no longer angry or depressed, he reaches a stage of resolution. Now he becomes less of a patient himself and more of a caregiver to his dog. It is at this point that healthcare information is best received.

If an owner has not really reached the acceptance stage, he may have negative reactions to caring for his dog. He may have difficulty remembering details about treatment. This is an important concept for both veterinary staff and the owners of newly diagnosed dogs.

As the acceptance stage is reached, it is valuable to consider this question: What are the "jobs" dogs do in this day and age?

With the exception of a few dogs that truly earn their keep as herding dogs, hunting dogs, or service dogs, most dogs today are generally unemployed. Our dogs have only a few basic functions in our homes. They alert us to visitors at the door. They want to cuddle in one form or another. And, they make us laugh. **Epileptic dogs can do all these things as well as other dogs.** They live relatively normal lives. Some epileptic, or "epi," dogs even have long and successful careers in obedience and agility sports.

While epilepsy will certainly have an effect on your dog, it is important to remember that current treatments are highly effective. The number of dogs successfully living with neurological disorders today confirms this. Appropriate treatment will reduce seizure activity and maintain the normal routine of daily living and recreation.

This book will give you the information and confidence to help you and your dog return to a sense of being "whole." You will regain a sense of control over your dog's health. With time, patience, and commitment, living with canine epilepsy will simply become part of your daily routine.

It is easy to think that you must be an instant expert — that you must know so many things at once. Learning about healthcare is more like a journey. Each day you will understand more about the problem and how your dog reacts. Turn to sections in the book that are most pressing to you now and read other sections as your schedule permits. Dealing with one thing at a time will help keep it all manageable.

As you progress with your dog's treatment, you may find yourselves bonding more closely. Giving medications and other treatments tends to deepen trust and improve communication. There is a special relationship that develops when you care for a dog with special needs.

It is also valuable, however, to keep balance in your life. Since epilepsy is a long-term condition, it's important for the caregiver to avoid burnout. Loss of sleep, stress, and worry can lead to feelings of exhaustion. Some owners may feel they cannot continue caring for an epileptic dog. These are normal emotions that are experienced by even the most compassionate people.

Be sure to take some time for relaxing activities. Many dogs sleep after seizures. If your schedule permits, take this opportunity to relax and regroup. Listen to soothing music or read a nice book. If you are losing sleep because your dog has seizures at night, or if you just need a break from your day-to-day worries, consider asking a trusted friend or family member to step in.

Children and Loss

Try to include children in the grieving process. Children often share a very strong bond to the family pet. Seizure activity can be especially frightening to them. They may experience feelings of anger and worry.

Including children in these painful times teaches them several things: That it is good to express emotion and fear and how to develop coping skills. As with yourself, give children permission to grieve.

Children can obviously sense when something is wrong. Avoiding the issue or lying about the dog's condition could result in lack of trust or irrational fear on the child's part. Adults who show respect for children's feelings help them build confidence in dealing with loss.

Openness and honesty encourage questions from the child. Straightforward answers are the best tactic. Be patient, as children may need to revisit issues repeatedly. Whenever appropriate, try to include all family members in the process of education and pet care.

References

Kubler-Ross, E., *On Death and Dying: What the Dying Have to Teach Doctors, Nurses, Clergy, and Their Own Families.* New York: Touchstone Books, 1969.

Chapter 2

The Doctor-Client Relationship

Optimum canine healthcare requires a trusting relationship between dog owner and veterinarian. Both parties must be active participants in the dog's care. Both must communicate effectively.

Several things contribute to the success of the relationship. These include the dog owner's learning style, his level of motivation, and the veterinarian's teaching style and experience. It is also helpful if the dog owner and doctor have shared philosophies about general healthcare issues.

The Veterinarian's Part

Some dog owners seek out the care of holistic veterinarians or veterinary specialists — veterinarians who specialize in the management of neurological disorders. Other owners have good experiences with their general-practice, hometown veterinarians. In these cases, the doctors do aggressive research to educate themselves and their clients. They are willing to consult with neurologists or more experienced veterinarians.

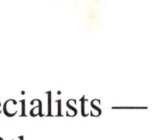

Other dog owners have poor results in this situation. They believe that doctors who are inexperienced in treating canine epilepsy are not current on the best therapies. Some owners become anxious that their dog's care is not as progressive as it could be. Since each dog will react differently to treatment, a doctor's level of experience can be a valuable asset.

To help decide this issue, many dog owners find it helpful to ask a few interview-type questions of the doctor. They want to know how many other epilepsy patients the doctor has (or is) treating, what treatments he employs, and how these pets have generally fared.

The veterinarian's practice style is another important element in a successful relationship. Some veterinarians may not be accustomed to including their clients as partners in the delivery of canine healthcare. Others are more forthcoming with their findings and opinions. They include the pet owner in discussions and decision-making.

Some brilliant clinicians, when faced with a hectic schedule, may appear brusque to clients. Most pet owners value bedside manner as much as technical competence. They want to feel comfortable asking questions of the doctor.

Finally, some doctors are simply better teachers than others. If a doctor does not explain things in a way that is understandable to each particular dog owner, it will not be helpful to the dog.

The Dog Owner's Part

Even the best veterinarian, however, cannot deliver effective care without the active participation of the dog owner. The owner must be willing to learn about his dog's condition and ask for clarification. He must accept his role as a caregiver. And, he must learn to assess the dog's condition, communicate this to the doctor, and make informed decisions.

Treatment Philosophies

There are two general approaches to caring for chronically ill dogs. In the first approach, veterinarians realize that caring for such pets can be a strain on families and can result in a sense of burnout. These doctors are concerned with keeping care simple and manageable for dog owners.

The second approach is a more aggressive one. It is usually pursued by people who want to do everything they can to maximize their dog's health. These are people who embrace the role of the caregiver and try to learn all they can about the disease.

Neither approach is wrong. Just as all dogs are different, so are their owners. People face many commitments in their lives: Professional, personal, family, and financial. What works in one family may not be a realistic option for another family. This book is written with both of these approaches in mind. It will offer a variety of options for you to consider and discuss with your veterinarian.

Dogs respond to treatment differently. While various standards do exist for such things as medication dosages, etc., individual dogs often respond outside these parameters. A good treatment plan will be flexible. It will take details into account that are particular to you and your dog.

In addition, it is important that the veterinarian and dog owner have a shared philosophy about basic dog care. Since treatment plans can include diet, exercise, acupuncture, medications, and supplements, it is important to have a doctor who will support your educated decisions and whatever strong beliefs you may have.

When there are glaring differences in these matters, it can be beneficial to seek a second opinion. (This is a very different scenario than the case of the dog owner in denial, searching for a miraculous cure.) Getting a second opinion is common in healthcare and most doctors are not insulted by it. Dog owners sometimes ask their friends for recommendations, or consult the telephone directory, veterinary-teaching hospital, or state veterinary association for a specialist or holistic practitioner.

A second opinion should also be sought when your veterinarian expresses hesitancy in treating your dog's epilepsy or perfunctorily instructs you to euthanize an otherwise healthy pet. A trusting, open relationship is vital to the successful treatment of your dog. He is a silent participant in all of this and you are his advocate.

Chapter 3

Normal Canine Structure and Function

To better understand seizure activity, it is helpful to examine the normal anatomy and function of the dog's body. This includes neural (nerve) function, endocrine (hormone) function, and metabolism. While this discussion may seem cumbersome at first, an understanding of these issues will become extremely helpful. The following brief descriptions are not intended to be comprehensive but rather prepare the reader for discussions yet to come.

The Gastrointestinal (GI) Tract

Since dogs do not chew their food but gulp it, instead, the **stomach** is the organ in which digestion actually begins. Unlike some other species, dogs do not have many of the molars needed to grind and mechanically break down food.

The **small intestine** is the portion of the gastrointestinal (GI) tract that follows the stomach. It is here that the majority of digestion occurs, including chemical breakdown and absorption of nutrients.

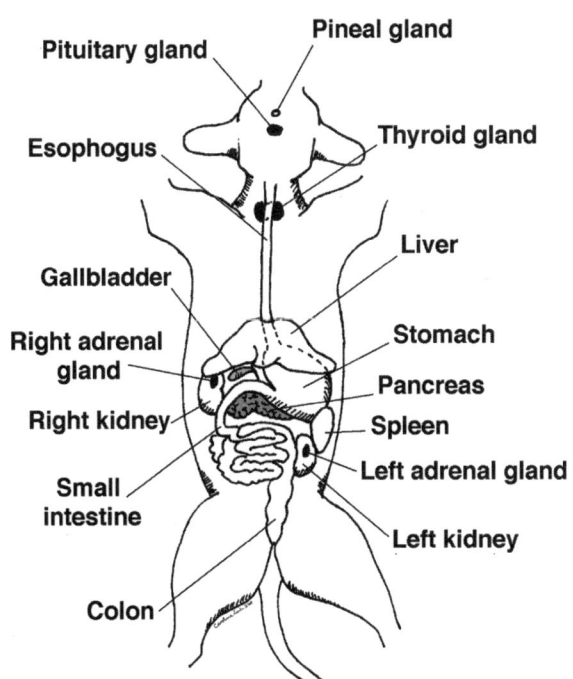

The **pancreas** is a glandular organ located in the abdomen, just below the stomach. It empties into the small intestine and is considered to be both a digestive organ and an endocrine gland. Accordingly, it has two distinct functions. One portion of the pancreas produces insulin. This portion is referred to as the **endocrine pancreas**. The other portion of the gland is called the **exocrine pancreas**. That portion produces digestive enzymes that help chemically break down food into useable nutrients.

The names of most enzymes end in the suffix "–ase." For example, **protease** digests proteins, **amylase** digests carbohydrates, and **lipase** digests fats (lipids). Digestive enzymes are secreted in a water-based solution. This solution flows into the small intestine via the pancreatic duct.

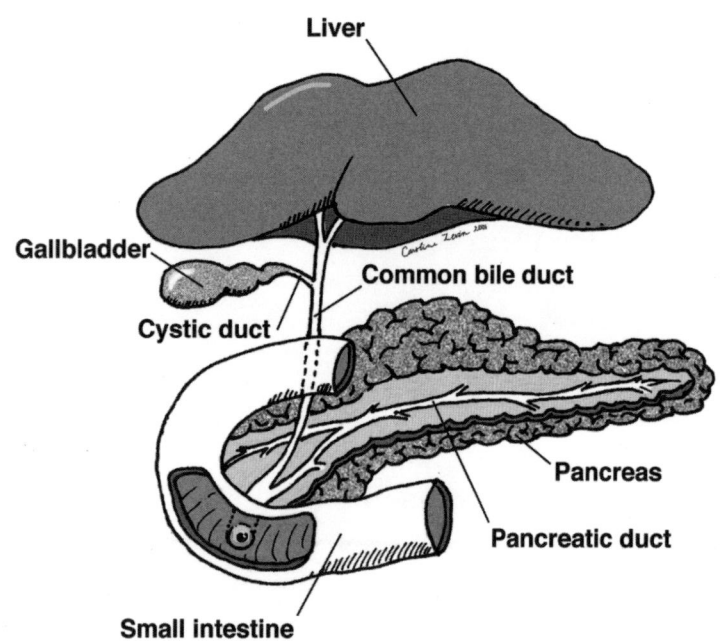

The **liver** is located alongside the stomach. It performs a multitude of jobs. It produces bile — a salty, yellowish fluid that plays an important part in the digestion of dietary fats. The liver is also the body's cleansing organ, modifying and detoxifying active substances in the bloodstream. These include hormones, medications, chemicals, and waste products such as bilirubin (a yellow pigment found in the bloodstream).

The **gallbladder** is situated alongside the liver. It functions as a storage tank for bile. When food enters the **small intestine**, the gallbladder secretes bile to help digest dietary lipids. En route to the small intestine, bile mixes with digestive enzymes in the common bile duct.

The **large intestine** is also referred to as the **colon**. It moves digested matter toward the rectum. One of its main functions is to reabsorb water from the GI tract, including the water that is secreted with digestive enzymes.

The **kidneys** adjust the chemical composition of the blood as necessary. The kidneys also filter the blood of poisons, chemicals, body wastes, and impurities. These impurities collect and concentrate in the dog's urine. They are excreted from the body when the dog urinates.

The Endocrine and Immune Systems

Located near the kidneys are two small endocrine glands known as the **adrenal glands**. These glands produce a number of natural hormones, including **cortisol**. Cortisol is a beneficial and crucial chemical in the healthy dog. It orchestrates a vast number of biological tasks in the body including metabolism and the immune-system response to stress and inflammation. It prepares the body for the fight-or-flight response and keeps the immune response in check. In normal cases, the adrenal glands secrete cortisol only as it is needed.

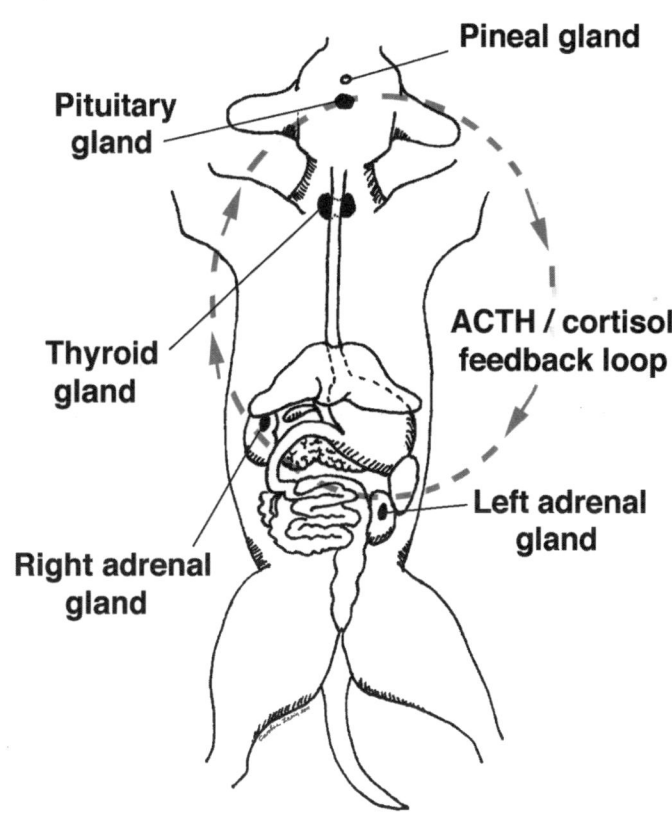

Cortisol secretion is controlled by another hormone called **adrenocorticotrophic hormone**, (also known as **ACTH**). ACTH is produced in the **pituitary**, an endocrine gland located at the base of the brain. When ACTH is released into the bloodstream, it stimulates the adrenal glands to release cortisol. Later, when the brain recognizes that sufficient levels of cortisol are present, the pituitary gland curtails the release of ACTH, which, in turn, halts the production of cortisol. This is known as a feedback loop.

Thyroid hormone is produced in the **thyroid gland,** located in the neck. This hormone regulates the body's metabolic rate (the rate at which cells burn oxygen and use nutrients), the quantity of energy the cells produce, and the number of enzymatic reactions that occur in the body. There are two main types of thyroid hormone: T4 and T3.

Reactions inside the thyroid gland cause iodine (a mineral) and tyrosine (an amino acid) to unite. When four iodine atoms bind with one tyrosine atom, the result is thyroxine hormone, also called **T4**, levo-thyroxine, or l-thyroxine. T4 is considered the "storage" or stored form of the hormone. Much of it is bound to protein molecules as it circulates through the bloodstream. You may hear this referred to as "bound T4." A smaller portion of T4 is not bound to protein. This is called "free T4."

Free T4 can be converted to the more active form of thyroid hormone, called **T3**. When T4 gives up one of its iodine atoms, it becomes T3 (also known as thyronine or triiodothyronine). A certain amount of T3 can be protein-bound as it circulates, but T3 is generally referred to as the *active* form of the hormone, which enters the cells and increases cellular metabolism.

Nestled behind the thyroid gland are the **parathyroid glands**. They produce **parathyroid hormone**, which, along with cortisol and kidney function, control calcium metabolism.

The **lymphatic system** is a network of tiny vessels that are similar to, but separate from, blood vessels. The lymphatic system produces many of the white blood cells needed to mount an immune response in the body. It also provides the entry route for dietary fats to enter the body.

Normal Canine Digestion and Metabolism

Every cell in the canine body requires a source of energy to live and work. Dogs eat a variety of fats, carbohydrates, and proteins to satisfy this need. Unlike the case in humans, the digestive process in dogs does not begin until food reaches the stomach. Here, strong hydrochloric acids begin to break apart the food. The stomach also secretes the enzyme pepsin, which begins the process of breaking down protein.

As food passes from the stomach into the small intestine, it stimulates the pancreas to release amylase, lipase, and protease. Up to this point, these enzymes have been inactive and stored in the pancreas. It is crucial that they remain inactive during storage since they might otherwise digest the pancreas itself (auto-digestion).

Digestive enzymes are released through the pancreatic duct to the small intestine. The pancreas also secretes an alkaline solution at this time. This solution provides the chemical environment necessary to activate the enzymes. Bile is simultaneously secreted by the gall bladder to aid in the digestion of lipids.

Carbohydrates

Amylase separates carbohydrates into smaller and smaller fragments with the result being **glucose**, a simple sugar molecule. It is the primary nutrient used by the brain and nervous system.

Glucose is transported from the digestive tract to the various cells in the body via the blood stream. The level of glucose in the bloodstream is referred to as **blood glucose** or **blood sugar**. Once the glucose molecules reach their destination, they must cross cell membranes to enter and nourish the cells. This crossing is accomplished with the help of **insulin,** a hormone produced by specialized beta cells (also known as islet cells) in the endocrine pancreas.

In normal dogs, the presence of glucose in the bloodstream stimulates the beta cells to produce a corresponding amount of insulin, which is then released into the bloodstream. When insulin molecules reach the various cells of the body, they attach to special areas on the cell walls known as receptors.

To illustrate this activity, imagine a hotel doorman holding open the door for his guests. Think of the hotel as the cell and the guest as the glucose. The doorman would play the role of insulin and the doorknob would be the receptor. The doorman allows the guests into the hotel much as **insulin allows passage of glucose into the cell.**

Once inside the cell, particularly a nerve cell, glucose is broken down further and triggers several other molecules to bind. One such molecule is adenosine. When adenosine combines with three phosphate molecules, the new molecule is called **adenosine triphosphate** (also known as **adenotriphosphate** or **ATP**). It functions as a source of power and energy for the cell. When energy is needed, one of the phosphate molecules "pops" off. This activity, called hydrolysis, releases energy.

The energy created from ATP hydrolysis helps transport small molecules across the membrane, assists in the synthesis of chemical compounds, and supports many other functions of cell life. Once ATP molecules release their energy, its pieces are later recycled to create new ATP molecules. All of these functions require adequate supplies of vitamins, minerals, oxygen, thyroid hormone, and glucose. Without sufficient thyroid activity and proper nutrients, the cell may not produce adequate energy.

The body maintains several protective, backup systems to ensure that the cells receive glucose. In the first system, the dog's body stores excess glucose for use at a later time. For example, just after mealtime, there is a great excess of glucose available — much more than the dog immediately needs. With the help of insulin, the body stores this excess glucose in the liver and various large muscles. This stored form of glucose is known as **glycogen**. When the cells become hungry, between meals and during sleep, the body can access glycogen.

The body can even create glucose from its own sources when food is not available. In cases of prolonged hunger, the body secretes **cortisol**, which tells the body to break down muscle protein (**catabolism**) or body fat (**lipolysis**) into glucose. In this way, cortisol ensures the presence of glucose in the bloodstream, providing energy for stressful times (the flight-or-fight response).

Finally, researchers believe that the body has some unique protective mechanisms that maintain a consistent environment in the brain. These mechanisms provide brain cells fairly constant levels of glucose and other nutrients. It does appear, however, that even this system can falter under chronically stressful situations.

Proteins

Dogs digest protein with a double dose of digestive enzymes. The stomach secretes pepsin and the pancreas secretes protease. If the system is working well, protein is broken down into very small chains of **amino acids**, the building blocks of all protein. To illustrate this concept, imagine a pearl necklace. The necklace itself is a dietary protein. Each individual pearl is an amino acid. To nourish the body, the necklace must be separated into small strands consisting of only a few pearls each.

Protein molecules perform a number of functions in the body. Proteins are the primary nutrients used to build and repair muscle tissue. They contribute to a host of normal body functions, including proper nerve and brain function. They form pores or **channels** through the nerve cell membranes. These channels allow nutrients and waste products to pass in and out of the cell. Other proteins, called identification proteins, are located in the cell membrane. These remind the immune system they "belong" to the body, distinguishing them from invading organisms. Insulin, thyroid hormone, various enzymes, and brain chemicals called **neurotransmitters** are all proteins.

Almost half of the amino acids required for life and wellness *must be supplied by diet*. These are called **essential amino acids** (**EAAs**). The body manufactures the remaining necessary amino acids from these. Those manufactured by the body are called **non-essential amino acids** (**NEAAs**). As with carbohydrate metabolism, the bloodstream transports protein fragments from the digestive tract to the various cells of the body.

Fats (Lipids)

Just as carbohydrates are broken down into simple sugars, and proteins are broken down into amino acids, dietary fats (or "lipids" to the nutritionist) are broken down into **fatty acids**. The digestion of dietary fats, however, is a little more complex than the digestion of other nutrients. This is because digestive enzymes are delivered to the small intestine in a solution of water. Since oil (fats) and water don't mix, the enzymes have difficulty attaching to the lipid molecules. If they cannot attach, they cannot break the molecular bonds.

To solve this problem, **bile** is secreted by the gallbladder. Bile salts act like laundry detergent, emulsifying lipid molecules. This process breaks down the lipid and exposes more surface to the effects of the digestive enzyme, lipase. Ultimately, short chains of fatty acids separate from this solution.

Bile salts are not normally excreted from the body. They are recycled. Once their work — emulsifying lipid molecules — is complete, they are reabsorbed from the intestine, recycled by the liver, and returned to the gallbladder for future use. This occurs through a closed system of blood vessels known as the portal system. Bile acid does not usually escape this system in a healthy dog.

The digestion of lipids takes one more odd turn. Instead of being absorbed directly into the blood stream, as are sugars and amino acids, fatty acids are taken up by the **lymphatic system**. Since the primary role of the lymphatic system is to fight infection, lipid digestion is really a secondary role to immune system function. Ultimately, however, lipids are dumped into the blood stream and circulated through the body. They provide a concentrated source of energy and comprise the basic structure of cell membranes.

Similar to essential amino acids (proteins), some fatty acids must be supplied by the diet. These are termed **essential fatty acids** or **EFAs**. Nutritionists classify EFAs into two main groups: Omega 3 fatty acids and Omega 6 fatty acids.

Omega 3 fatty acids, such as Docosahexaenoic acid (DHA), are generally found in fish oils, some vegetables, and vegetable oils. **Omega 6 fatty acids**, such as Gamma-Linoleic Acid (GLA) are more common in the diet and found in animal fat and vegetables. Both play a large role in normal brain function. They are necessary to produce **phospholipids**, molecules that provide the framework of brain cell membranes. When membranes contain an appropriate amount of phospholipids, they remain fluid and flexible. Nutrients and wastes can easily pass through the walls of such cells.

Some Other Important Nutrients

An intimate relationship exists between the immune system, hormone production, and dietary vitamins and minerals. **Sodium, potassium**, and **chloride** regulate body pH and fluid balance in the body. **Phosphorus** is found in many types of cell membranes and is intricately involved with cell metabolism and ATP energy production. **Calcium** is required for dental and skeletal bone strength. It also plays a role in nerve conduction, muscle contraction, and glandular secretions.

Once inside the tissues of the body, these substances take on electrical charges and are termed **ions**. Sodium (abbreviated $Na+$), potassium ($K+$), and calcium ($Ca2+$) all carry a positive electrical charge. Chloride ($Cl-$) carries a negative charge. Ions are deeply involved with nerve transmissions.

Magnesium is necessary for a vast number of biochemical processes including metabolism, energy production (ATP hydrolysis), muscle relaxation, and nervous system function. Magnesium activates more than 75% of metabolic enzymes in the body, including the enzyme reactions that build necessary neurotransmitters and dispose of cellular waste products. Magnesium helps maintain sodium and potassium balance. This relationship is essential to normal water balance in the body. The presence of magnesium is required for calcium to be deposited into skeletal bone, cartilage, and ligaments.

Vitamin E and **Vitamin A** are necessary for normal vision and peripheral nervous system function. These, in addition to **Vitamin C,** play important roles in supporting immune system function. The **B vitamins**, particularly B6 or pyridoxine, are necessary for the body to produce calming brain chemicals, such as **gamma-aminobutyric acid** (or **GABA**).

As nutrients are broken down by normal metabolism, molecules called **free radicals** result. Free radicals are unstable molecules with one unpaired electron. These molecules travel through the body searching for another electron with which to pair. Eventually, free radicals are able to find and steal an electron from a stable molecule somewhere in the body's cells. This leaves the second molecule weakened or unstable, damaging cell structures, including cell membranes. This process is called **oxidation**. Vitamins A, C, and E have antioxidant properties, soaking up free radicals, and protecting membranes from their damage.

In addition to causing membrane damage, free radicals also inhibit a crucial function of metabolism. They inhibit a process known as the **activated methyl cycle**. This is a chemical process that occurs when one molecule of adenosine (donated from the ATP molecule) pops off and combines with methionine, one of the essential amino acids. This process occurs with the help of magnesium and creates a compound called **S-adenosylmethionine** (or **SAMe**). SAMe contains "methyl groups," molecules made of carbon and hydrogen atoms. When needed, these methyl groups break off from the SAMe molecule and start other chemical and enzyme reactions in the body. This process is known as **methylation.**

Methylation is responsible for building thousands of chemicals and hormones necessary for normal body function. It produces **melatonin** (the sleep inducing hormone) from serotonin (the "feel good" brain chemical). Methylation produces gamma-aminobutyric acid or **GABA**, (the calming brain chemical). Methylation transfers metabolic wastes from the brain. And methylation is intricately involved with the process of **genetic expression**—how genes work.

When SAMe donates its methyl group for such chemical reactions, it also creates a by-product. This is the chemical **homocysteine**. Normally, homocysteine is recycled. It combines with certain B vitamins and magnesium to recreate methionine and the whole process begins again.

Vitamin D assists the pancreas to produce insulin and helps the immune system differentiate between friend and foe (self and non-self). It also orchestrates the process of calcium absorption.

When Vitamin D enters the body, it is considered inactive. Processes that occur in the kidneys and the liver activate it. Once activated, it is called **Vitamin D hormone**. Vitamin D hormone regulates serum levels of calcium by pulling it from the diet or from skeletal bone. The kidney's production rate of active Vitamin D, in turn, is regulated by parathyroid hormone.

The Brain

The brain is comprised of numerous structures that control both voluntary and involuntary activities in the body. The brain constitutes only a small portion of the body's weight, yet requires 20% of the body's available oxygen, and a *continuous* supply of oxygen, at that. In addition to oxygen, brain cells require a constant supply of glucose from the bloodstream.

The largest section of the brain is the **cerebrum**. It is divided into two hemispheres—right and left — which are further divided into lobes. The **frontal lobe** is the area located behind the dog's forehead. This portion of the brain is believed to control motor function. The **temporal lobes** are located laterally (to the sides) of the frontal lobe, near the temples. Temporal lobe function includes auditory (hearing) and vocal behavior. At the top of the brain, located just under the crown of the skull, is the **parietal lobe**. This area of the brain is responsible for sensory behavior. Finally, there is the **occipital lobe**, located at the back of the head. The occipital lobe regulates visual behavior.

Other structures in the brain include the midbrain, brainstem, hypothalamus, and cerebellum. These areas combine with frontal lobe activity to regulate emotional behavior. The brain also houses several endocrine glands that produce important hormones.

The **midbrain** and **brainstem** are structures that transition the brain to the spinal cord. The **hypothalamus** controls pituitary gland function. All are involved with more basic activities of life. This includes heart and respiratory rate, hunger, thirst, sleep, and temperature control. Unlike human anatomy, these structures extend into the neck of the dog.

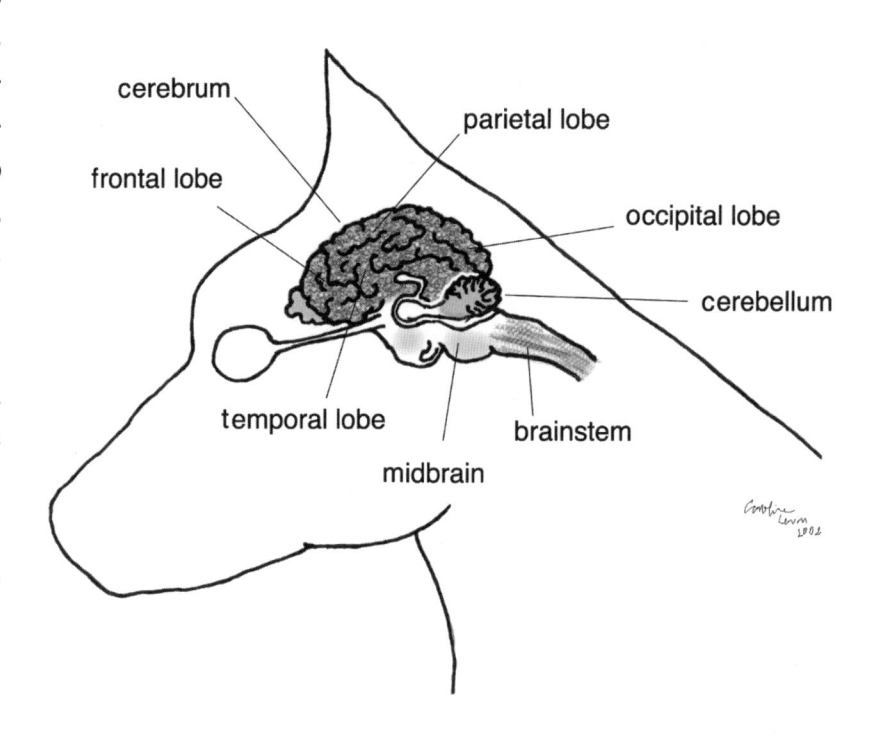

The **pituitary gland**, located deep within the brain, is a master gland of the endocrine (hormone) system. It produces important hormones that "talk to" other glands in the body. For example, the pituitary gland produces adrenocorticotrophic hormone (ACTH) and thyroid stimulating hormone (TSH), among others. ACTH stimulates the adrenal glands, and TSH stimulates the thyroid gland.

Another important endocrine gland located within the brain is the **pineal gland**. This small gland is responsible for maintaining daily wake/sleep cycles known as circadian rhythms. The pineal gland accomplishes this by releasing the hormone **melatonin** as evening falls.

Such hormones exhibit a complex relationship with the immune system and brain function. So important is this relationship that entirely new fields of medicine have recently evolved around it. Neuroimmunology examines the connection between the brain and the immune system. Neuroendocrinology examines the link between the brain and the body's hormones. Dog lovers, too, are starting to recognize these connections.

The **cerebellum** is a small, cauliflower-shaped structure located between the cerebrum and the midbrain/brainstem. The cerebellum is involved with balance and coordination. It integrates the nerve pathways of the brain to maintain organized motor function (muscle movement).

The brain is suspended in a solution called **cerebrospinal fluid (CSF)**. This acts as both a cushion and a nutrient source for brain tissue. CSF flows around the outside of the brain, as well as through internal cavities, called **ventricles.**

The brain protects itself with a defense mechanism known as the **blood-brain barrier**, a combination of membranes and tightly packed cells that line the blood vessels of the brain. This barrier maintains the delicate balance of oxygen and glucose required by brain cells and protects them from the effects of toxins and many medications. Medications for neurological illnesses must be specially formulated to pass through this barrier in order to reach the brain.

The brain is comprised of two main types of cells. **Neurons** are the cells that form a network of electrical pathways, communicate with each other, and send messages to muscles and organs of the body. **Glial cells** provide a supportive framework for neurons and regulate the concentration of certain chemicals in the brain.

Neurons

Each neuron is shaped a little bit like a starfish. The central body of the neuron contains the cell **nucleus** and **mitochondria**, the tiny structures that produce energy (ATP production). They are the power plants of the cell.

Stretching out from the cell body are multitudes of arms known as **dendrites**. Most dendrites are designed to *receive* the messages from other neurons. (Each neuron can conceivably be in contact with thousands of other neurons throughout the brain.) Each neuron also has one specialized, elongated arm known as an **axon**. The axon terminates in tiny bulbs known as **telodendrites**. This arm is designed to *send* messages to other cells.

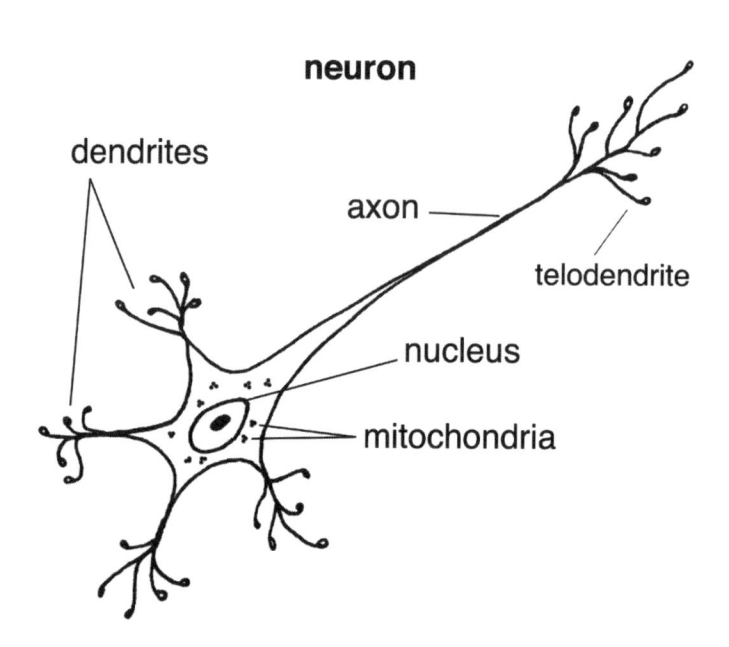

Cell Membranes

The cell membrane, a thin structure that encases each neuron, is receiving increasing attention from epilepsy researchers. It plays a vital role in how the cell nourishes itself, repairs itself, and generates electrical impulses. The content and effectiveness of cell membranes change from moment to moment due to the effects of diet, stressors, and immune system messengers. Even a slight alteration in the membrane can have a negative affect on the ability of a neuron to work effectively.

The cell membrane is basically comprised of a double row of **phospholipids**. Phospholipid molecules consist of fatty acid chains attached to phosphoglyceride heads. The membrane is normally semi-permeable, allowing small particles to pass in and out of the cell. These particles include nutrients, waste products, and ions such as sodium (Na+), potassium (K+), chloride (Cl-), and calcium (Ca2+).

Normally, concentrations of potassium are high *inside* the cell, while concentrations of sodium, chloride, and calcium are higher in the fluid that *surrounds* the cell. The net result is that the inside of the cell carries a negative electrical charge, while the outside of the cell carries a positive electrical charge.

Receptors

Embedded in the phospholipid membrane are a variety of protein molecules. Some proteins stud the interior or the exterior of the membrane. The latter can act as receptors, which allow neurotransmitters and hormones to bind to the membrane and receive entrance into the cell. A single neuron can have several types of receptors. For example, some receptors receive hormones such as thyroid or insulin. Some receive messages that calm the cell. Other receptors receive messages that stimulate the cell.

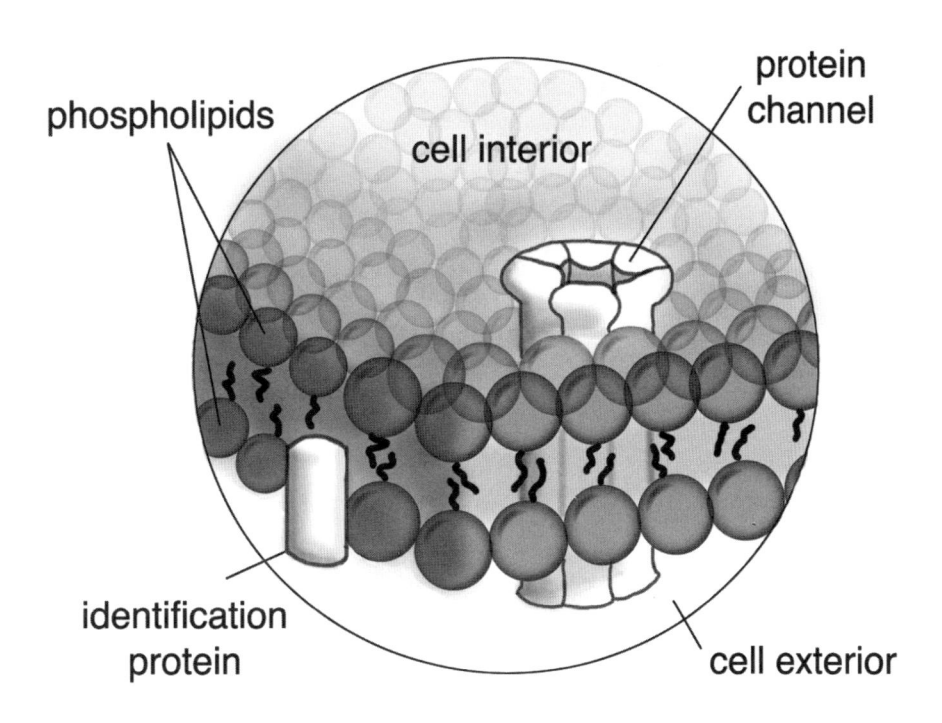

Channels

Certain protein molecules protrude through *both* sides of the cell membrane. When clustered together, they form channels or portals of entry in to the cell. Ions move in and out of the cell in various ways. In some cases, channels are continuously open. In other cases, the channels are "gated" and only open with an electrical signal (voltage).

Normal Nerve Transmission

Neurons communicate with each other by a fascinating method of electrical and chemical messengers. The messengers that travel between neurons are chemicals called **neurotransmitters** (**NTs**). In normal dogs, the levels of these chemicals are carefully balanced, producing normal mental and physical function.

Scientists have identified as many as 50 neurotransmitters. Some sources define them as protein molecules (amino acids) and other sources define them as hormones. Regardless of the nomenclature, NTs are key to normal nerve cell transmissions — the rapid exchange of chemicals and electrical currents.

Neurotransmitters are released from storage vesicles at the end of a cell's axon (the telodendrites). The neurotransmitters then travel across a microscopic space known as a **synapse** and connect with receptors on the adjacent cell. Once the NT connects with its receptor, it will cause a specific reaction to occur in the cell. For our purposes, we will limit our discussion to two main types of neurotransmitters: Those that calm a cell (**inhibitory NTs**) and those that stimulate a cell (**excitatory NTs**).

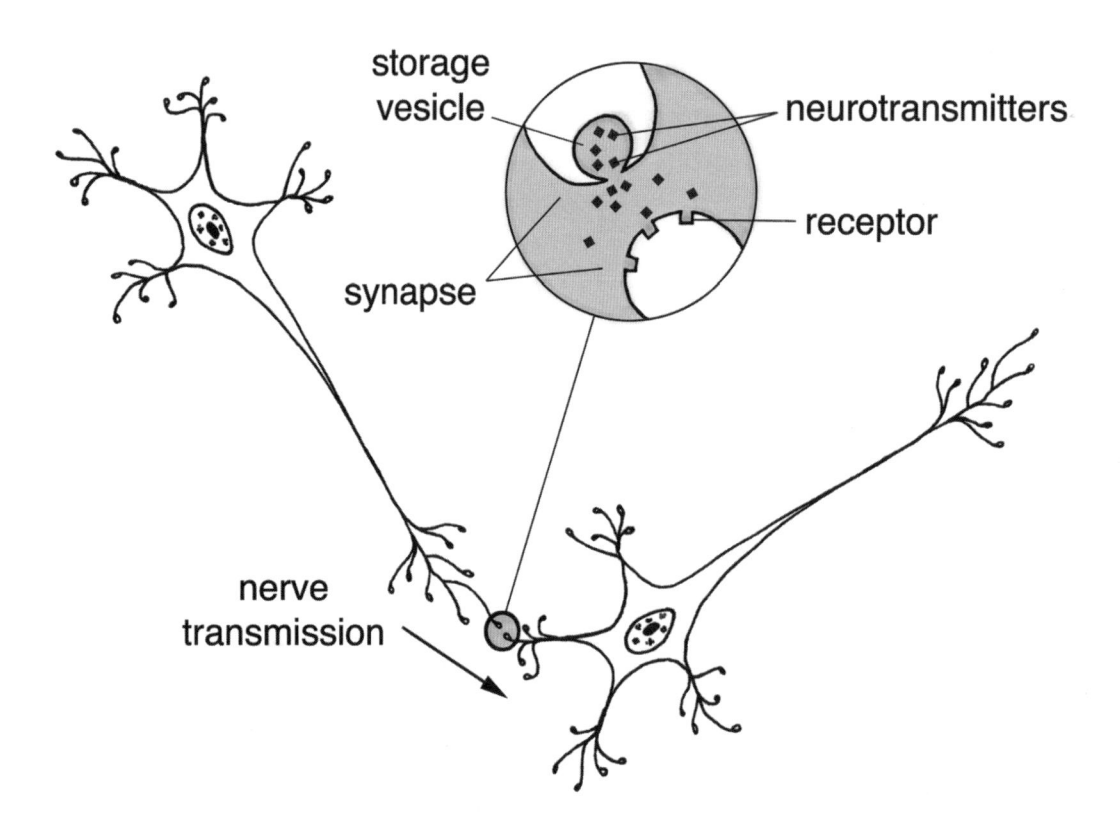

If a large volume of excitatory NTs, such as **glutamate** or **aspartate**, bind with a large number of excitatory receptors, the following reaction will occur. Protein channels (pores) in the cell membrane will open for a fraction of a second. During that time, potassium (K+) will leave the cell and sodium (Na+) will rush into the cell. This process will be repeated down the length of the membrane. In the end, the cell will have a *positive charge on the inside* and a negative charge on the outside. This is an abrupt change from the cell's normal resting state and has the effect of creating an electrical current. This is often described as a neuron **firing**.

When this electrical current passes down the length of the axon and reaches the telodendrite, the cycle is repeated. Neurotransmitters are released, cross the synapse, and cause the next neuron to fire. This continues until the NTs finally reach the cells of a muscle. When the transmission reaches the muscle, contractions occur. The results are such movements as walking, scratching, breathing, etc.

Nerve cell transmissions are not limited to excitatory firing, however. Some nerve cell transmissions are actually calming or inhibiting reactions. In these cases, a large number of inhibitory NTs, such as **gamma-aminobutyric acid** (**GABA**) or **glycine**, bind with a large number of inhibitory receptors. A different set of membrane channels open. These channels allow chloride (Cl-) ions into the cell, while potassium (K+) ions move out. The net result is that the inside of the cell has a *very negative* charge or becomes **hyperpolarized**. In fact, the cell is so negatively charged, that it will not fire. In this case the "reaction" the neurotransmitters cause is that of actually keeping the adjacent cell *still*.

If more excitatory NTs reach their respective receptors than do inhibitory NTs, the cell will likely fire, and vice versa. This relationship explains why you can sit quietly and read this book, without having your arms and legs flail about. Daily life consists of a constant balance between certain neurons firing while others are inhibited. It is a process that requires a great deal of cellular energy from the combined efforts of ATP, oxygen, glucose, and other nutrients.

NOTE: Interestingly, both GABA (the inhibitory NT) and glutamate (the excitatory NT) stem from the same amino acid: **Glutamic acid**. The main difference in their metabolism is that glutamic acid is first converted to gluta*mine* before being converted to GABA. Vitamin B6 (pyridoxine) and SAMe play a role in this conversion.

After firing, a neuron must return to its resting state, that of being negatively charged. To achieve this, sodium molecules (Na+) must be moved out of the cell and potassium (K+)

must be allowed back in. The hydrolysis of ATP molecules provides the energy to carry out this activity. You may hear this referred to as the sodium-potassium pump. This exchange leaves the cell with a slightly negative charge and the surrounding fluid with a positive charge. In this state, the cell is ready to receive new nerve transmissions and react accordingly.

References

Bourre, J.M., *Brainfood: A Provocative Exploration of the Connection Between What You Eat and How You Think*. Boston: Little, Brown and Company, 1998.

Carlson, D.G., and Giffin, J.M., *Dog Owner's Home Veterinary Handbook*. New York: Howell Book House, 1992.

Clemmons, R.M., "Clinical Neurology in a Nutshell," http:// pawcare.com/rclemmons, 2002.

Frankel, P., and Madsen, F., *Stop Homocysteine Through the Methylation Process*. Thousand Oaks, CA: TRC Publications, 1998.

Ganong, W.F., *Review of Medical Physiology*. Norwalk, CT: Appleton & Lange, 1993.

Levin, C.D., *Dogs, Diet and Disease: An Owner's Guide to Diabetes Mellitus, Pancreatitis, Cushing's Disease, and More*. Oregon City: Lantern Publications, 2001.

Lombard, J., and Germano, C., *The Brain Wellness Plan*. New York: Kensington Publishing Corporation, 1998.

National Institute of Neurological Disorders: "Seizures and Epilepsy," http://www.ninds.nih.gov/health_and_medical/pbs/seizures_and_epilepsy_htr.htm, 2001.

Osiecki, H., *The Physician's Handbook of Clinical Nutrition*. Kelvin Grove, Australia: Bio Concepts Publishing, 1995.

Richard, A., and Reiter, J., *Epilepsy: A New Approach*. New York: Prentice Hall, 1990.

Shames, R., and Shames K.H., *Thyroid Power: Ten Steps to Total Health*. New York: Harper Resource, 2001.

Chapter 4

Epilepsy: Definitions and Diagnosis

In the epileptic dog, the brain and body do not function as described in Chapter 3. Instead, there are chemical imbalances or alterations in how the brain is "wired." Neurons do not connect and communicate with each other in the normal way. Consequently, the careful balance between excitation and inhibition is disturbed.

Scientists believe that epileptics experience an excess of excitatory neurotransmissions or insufficient inhibitory neurotransmissions. Either situation can result in too much neuronal activity. Thousands, or perhaps, millions, of neurons discharge simultaneously and for prolonged periods. These dogs may experience strange sensations, behaviors, and muscle spasms. Consequently, the condition of epilepsy is sometimes described as an electrical storm.

Defining Epilepsy

Defining epilepsy is nearly a science unto itself. Various sources and veterinarians use terminology quite differently. Epilepsy cases can be classified in several ways — by the *cause of the problem* or the *type* of seizure. However, as we examine the everyday influences faced by companion dogs (diet, vaccines, and chemicals), the various classifications of epilepsy begin to blur. The links between diet, metabolism, hormones, immunity, and genetics are so intricate that they will be examined separately in Chapter 5, *Seizure-provoking Factors*.

Epilepsy Classified by Cause

Idiopathic/Genetic Causes

If an epilepsy case has an unknown cause, it is defined as **idiopathic** epilepsy. Some sources also define this as **inherited** or **primary** epilepsy. This is the type most commonly diagnosed in dogs. These dogs are suspected to have an inborn biochemical defect of the neurons in the brain. In some breeds, the onset of idiopathic epilepsy often occurs between six months and five years of age.

Patterns of genetic epilepsy are not clear to breeders and scientists. The mode of transmission may differ between various breeds. In some breeds, it appears that transmission may involve more than one gene or multiple areas on a gene, making it difficult to predict the outcome of a particular breeding.

Veterinarians strongly suspect a genetic tendency in the following breeds of dogs: Beagle, Belgian Tervuren, Dachshund, German Shepherd Dog, and Keeshond. Additionally, the following breeds demonstrate a higher than average rate of seizures, which may also indicate a genetic tendency: Akita, Border Collie, Bouvier, Boxer, Cocker Spaniel, Collie, Dalmatian, Golden Retriever, Irish Setter, Labrador Retriever, Miniature Schnauzer, Norwich Terrier, Poodle, Siberian Husky, St. Bernard, and Wire Fox Terrier.

In other cases, the epilepsy may have a **known cause.** Some sources do not consider these to be true cases of epilepsy, but rather, **seizure disorders**. The seizures are secondary to, and merely part of, some larger problem. Below are some examples.

Developmental Causes

Abnormalities in brain wiring (nerve connections) may occur during brain development. **Hydrocephalus**, a condition in which excess cerebrospinal fluid (CSF) accumulates in the brain, is one of these developmental problems. The body may produce excess CSF, poorly reabsorb it, or block the normal flow. These scenarios cause excess pressure on brain tissue and abnormal wiring of brain cells. The following breeds are prone to hydrocephalus: Boston Terrier, Chihuahua, English Bulldog, Lhasa Apso, Maltese, Miniature Pinscher, Pekingese, Pomeranian, Pug, Toy Poodle, and Yorkshire Terrier.

Other congenital, structural deformities can also cause seizures. This includes deformities of brain tissue, as well as birth defects elsewhere in the body. One of these is a portacaval or **portosystemic shunt**, a condition in which veins return blood to the general circulation before it has been cleansed by the liver. Unfiltered by the liver, this blood recirculates waste products and chemicals through the body. Maltese, Miniature Schnauzers, and Yorkshire Terriers are prone to congenital portosystemic shunts. In addition, other breeds may develop shunts in response to liver disease that develops later in life.

Nutritional/Metabolic Causes

Altered nerve cell function may stem from **vitamin deficiency** (specifically the B vitamins), or **hypoglycemia** (low blood sugar). Rhyme "hypo" with "low" to remember the meaning. Altered levels of calcium can contribute to seizures. **Hypocalcemia** can result from insufficient parathyroid gland function and chronic renal failure. **Hypercalcemia** is also believed to contribute to chronic renal failure.

In some epileptic dogs, there appears to be a connection between seizure activity and insufficient **thyroid hormone**. While this is the source of some debate in the veterinary community, a number of dog owners report a reduction in seizures following the administration of prescription thyroid hormone. The correlation may involve the fact that thyroid hormone controls the rate of metabolism, energy production, and other normal functions inside brain cells and on the membranes.

In other cases, neural cell metabolism is altered due to missing enzymes. Normally, various enzymes break down metabolic waste products. However, in some dogs, these enzymes are deficient. Without them, waste products do not break down. Instead, they accumulate in the cell, impinging on normal cell function and health. You may hear this referred to as a **storage disease** or a degenerative disease. These dogs are born with normal cell metabolism (enzyme function) which later degenerates as the dog ages.

The list of breeds affected by storage diseases is long. It includes: Australian Cattle Dog, Basset Hound, Beagle, Blue Heeler, Border Collie, Cairn Terrier, Chihuahua, Cocker Spaniel, Coonhound, Dachshund, English Setter, German Shorthaired Pointer, Japanese Spaniel, Miniature Pincher, Miniature Poodle, Pomeranian, Portuguese Water Dog, Saluki, Springer Spaniel, Tibetan Terrier, West Highland White Terrier, and mixed-breed dogs.

Finally, in dogs with impaired kidney function, waste products such as **uremic acid** — a product of protein metabolism — may not be adequately cleansed from the bloodstream. As these waste products are recycled through the system (uremia), seizures may result.

Kidney degeneration can also cause altered electrolyte levels. This includes alterations in calcium and potassium levels, both of which are important to normal nerve conduction.

Additional Causes: Trauma, Tumors, Strokes, Hypoxia, and More

Scientists believe that following a **stroke** or **injury**, the body's attempt to repair itself may inadvertently result in abnormal nerve connections. These abnormal connections are believed to cause epilepsy. Some dogs experience seizures after being hit by a car, a baseball, or suffering physical abuse. Sharp collar corrections applied at the base of the neck may also be harmful. Seizure onset usually occurs by six months to one year after the injury and may last for weeks to years.

Events that deprive the brain of oxygen (**hypoxia**) can damage neurons and also contribute to epilepsy. Examples of this include: Near-drowning, cardiac problems (murmurs, congestive heart failure), stroke, or insufficient oxygen at the time of birth.

Brain **tumors** can cause seizures. The neurons surrounding the tumor cells may be compressed, distorted, or hypoxic. In some cases, seizures precede the diagnosis of a tumor. This is because the tumor may be small or difficult to see on imaging tests. Seizures may worsen as the tumor grows. The following breeds are prone to various types of tumors: Boston Terrier, Boxer, Collie, English Bulldog, and German Shepherd Dog. The risk of tumors generally increases with age.

Other sources of seizures include hyperthermia (fever, hot-weather exercise), infection (tick-borne diseases such as ehrlichoisis and Rocky Mountain spotted fever), inflammation/swelling (encephalitis, meningitis), brain parasites, toxins, pesticides, and poisons. These cases are not always considered true epilepsy if seizures resolve themselves. Epilepsy or seizure disorders are usually diagnosed after the patient has had two or more seizures.

Epilepsy Classified by Seizure Type

Seizure terminology has undergone changes in recent years. The new terminology describes whether the electrical discharge occurs on both sides of the brain (a generalized seizure) or in just part of the brain (a partial seizure.) Below are definitions of the most current terminology.

Generalized Seizures

These terms refer to seizures in which *most* of the neurons in the brain discharge simultaneously. Generalized seizures are frequently preceded by an unusual sensation, called an aura, and are the most common seizures diagnosed in dogs. Symptoms may include: Stiffening (the tonic phase) and/or jerking of the entire body (the clonic phase.) These dogs may collapse, snap their jaws, salivate, howl, lose bladder or bowel control, empty their anal sacs, lose consciousness, or even stop breathing. This type of seizure was previously termed Grand Mal, which means "big badness."

Some dogs may remain conscious during all of this. Others may have a blank appearance. These seizures are sometimes referred to as "absence" seizures since the patient appears to be lost in thought or mentally absent for a few moments. (Occasionally, absence seizures are classified under the heading of "partial" seizures.) Absence seizures are not commonly diagnosed in dogs.

Typically, when the dog relaxes and becomes limp, the seizure is over. Since generalized seizures involve most of the brain, these dogs may also experience some of the other symptoms listed below. Specifically, this can include mood and memory changes seen in complex partial seizures.

Partial Seizures or Focal Seizures

These terms refer to seizures in which only *a portion* of the neurons discharge. Typically the disturbance is confined to one area or part of the brain. You may hear these types of seizures described by their location, such as temporal lobe epilepsy or frontal lobe epilepsy, for example. Terms such as these describe the area where the seizure originates, also known as the seizure **focus**. The neurons in surrounding areas are able to prevent excessive firing. However, in some cases, partial seizures can develop into generalized seizures.

Partial Seizures or Focal Seizures (con't)

Complex partial seizures are those partial seizures in which the dog experiences a change in, or loss of, consciousness. Complex partial seizures may include snapping, chewing, or licking motions. These seizures tend to involve portions of the brain that regulate emotion and memory. Seizure activity can be reflected by alterations in fear, confusion, or aggression. If the seizure includes areas of the brain involved with memory, a dog may not recognize familiar people and places. He may growl at family members until completely recovered or may feel the need to reintroduce himself once the seizure is over. This type of seizure may also cause alterations in vision, even hallucinations of imaginary flies.

Simple partial seizures are those in which there is no change in consciousness but include the stiffening or jerking of a small part of the body. Some dogs turn their head in an unusual way. Some may blink or twitch.

In some cases, the area of excessive discharge is so small, that the dog may only demonstrate minor outward effects or **aura** behaviors. The nature of the aura is often similar from one episode to the next and symptoms are indicative of the part of the brain involved. Auras commonly include feelings of intense fear, dizziness, irritability, or unease. Some dogs may have dilated pupils or their eyes may lose focus. An aura *may* develop into a more involved seizure if the discharge activity spreads to a larger area of the brain.

Cluster Seizures

This term refers to the phenomenon of seizures occurring close together, over a period of several days or hours. This can entail generalized or partial seizures. Generalized cluster seizures can lead to a more serious condition called status epilepticus.

Status Epilepticus

This is a scenario in which seizures occur continuously for more than five minutes, or those that occur one after another. During status epilepticus, the dog may not fully regain consciousness between seizures. These repeated seizures can interfere with normal breathing and heart function, resulting in hypoxia (insufficient oxygen) to the brain. Irreversible brain and organ damage — and even death — can occur. Status epilepticus is considered an emergency situation and requires immediate veterinary care. This may include sedation and IV fluids at the veterinary clinic.

Diagnosing Epilepsy

Your veterinarian will perform a number of examinations and tests prior to making the diagnosis of epilepsy. Such a work-up includes a physical and neurological examination. The neurological exam evaluates reflexes, sensations, gait, and the function of the cranial nerves (the 12 pairs of nerves that emanate directly from the brain). This exam can assist the doctor in identifying the location of an underlying lesion such as a tumor or other physical damage.

Blood samples help screen for metabolic disorders that may be associated with seizures. They may also identify infections, lead poisoning, or concurrent illnesses such as diabetes, altered liver function, or anemia. Urine and fecal tests may also be ordered.

> **Laboratory tests** may include:
> Complete blood count (CBC)
> Chemistry profile
> Serum cholinesterase
> Serum bile acid concentrations
> Urinalysis
> Blood glucose testing
> Serum lead levels
> Parasite examinations

In the case of idiopathic epilepsy, many if not all of these laboratory tests may have normal results since the inborn defect does not cause abnormalities except during the seizure. In cases of acquired epilepsy, findings may be abnormal. This distinguishes them from cases of idiopathic epilepsy. Your veterinarian may also recommend one or more of the imaging tests listed below.

Electroencephalogram (EEG)

This procedure creates a pen and ink tracing or digital image of the brain's electrical activity. Dogs are usually lightly sedated for this procedure. Electrodes (similar to EKG patches) that measure the electrical potential of the brain are attached to the scalp. Doctors look for abnormal patterns in the brain waves. EEG results can be inconclusive in diagnosing epilepsy since brain activity may appear normal between seizures.

Computerized Axial Tomography (CAT) Scan

A CAT scan provides images of the brain that can help doctors diagnose tumors, strokes, or brain atrophy. Dogs are usually fasted and anesthetized for this procedure. Unfortunately, for diagnostic purposes, the result is often normal in epileptic individuals.

Magnetic Resonance Imaging (MRI)

This procedure utilizes a magnetic field, radio waves, and a computer (but no radiation) to produce a detailed image of brain anatomy. Dogs are usually anesthetized for this procedure. This image can provide information on structural problems, including soft tissue and blood vessel anatomy.

Spinal Tap

A spinal tap is performed under general anesthesia, as well, and involves aspirating and culturing a small amount of cerebrospinal fluid (CSF). This can be helpful in identifying cases of infection, such as meningitis.

Radiograph (x-rays)

X-rays may be helpful in identifying skeletal deformities.

References

Carlson, D.G., and Giffin, J.M., *Dog Owner's Home Veterinary Handbook*. New York: Howell Book House, 1992.

Clemmons, R.M., "Clinical Neurology in a Nutshell," http:// pawcare.com/rclemmons, 2002.

Crook, A., Dawson, S., and Hill, B., "Globoid Cell Leukodystrophy," *Canine Inherited Disease Database*, Atlantic Veterinary College, University of Prince Edward Island, http://www.upei.ca/~cidd/: 2001

National Institute of Neurological Disorders: "Seizures and Epilepsy," http://www.ninds.nih.gov/health_and_medical/pbs/seizures_and_epilepsy_htr.htm, 2001.

Oliver, J.E., Lorenz, M.D., and Kornegay, J.N., *Handbook of Veterinary Neurology, Third Edition*. Philadelphia: WB Saunders Company, 1997.

Richard, A., and Reiter, J., *Epilepsy: A New Approach*. New York: Prentice Hall, 1990.

Canine Epilepsy

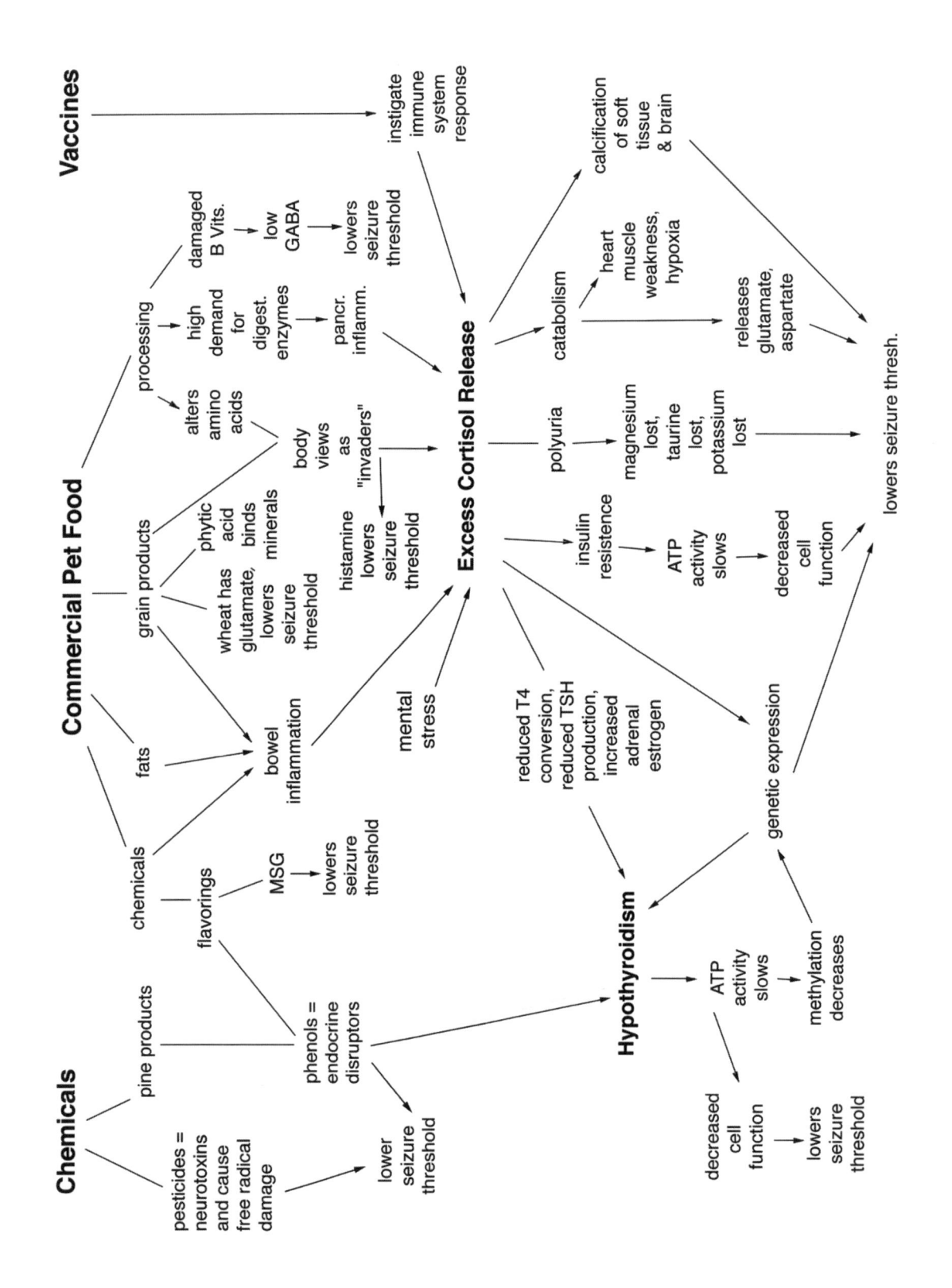

Vaccines → instigate immune system response

Commercial Pet Food
- processing → damaged B Vits. → low GABA → lowers seizure threshold
- processing → high demand for digest. enzymes → pancr. inflamm.
- processing → alters amino acids → body views as "invaders" → Excess Cortisol Release
- grain products → phytic acid binds minerals
- grain products → wheat has glutamate, lowers seizure threshold
- grain products → histamine lowers seizure threshold
- fats → bowel inflammation
- chemicals → bowel inflammation
- flavorings → MSG → lowers seizure threshold
- flavorings → phenols = endocrine disruptors → lower seizure threshold
- phenols → Hypothyroidism

Chemicals
- pine products → phenols = endocrine disruptors
- pesticides = neurotoxins and cause free radical damage → lower seizure threshold

bowel inflammation → body views as "invaders"
mental stress → Excess Cortisol Release

Excess Cortisol Release
- → calcification of soft tissue & brain
- → catabolism → heart muscle weakness, hypoxia → releases glutamate, aspartate → calcification of soft tissue & brain
- → releases glutamate, aspartate → lowers seizure thresh.
- → polyuria → magnesium lost, taurine lost, potassium lost → lowers seizure thresh.
- → insulin resistence → ATP activity slows → decreased cell function → lowers seizure thresh.
- → reduced T4 conversion, reduced TSH production, increased adrenal estrogen → Hypothyroidism
- → genetic expression

Hypothyroidism
- → ATP activity slows → decreased cell function → lowers seizure threshold
- → methylation decreases → genetic expression → Excess Cortisol Release

Chapter 5

Seizure-provoking Factors

Unlike in years past, today's dogs are routinely exposed to increasing numbers of chemicals and commercial products. Such factors demonstrate highly suspicious connections to epilepsy. This chapter will examine each of these topics.

Part I: Diet

Life is more hectic, urban, and commercial than it was 30 or 40 years ago. This has clearly been reflected in how we feed ourselves and our dogs. We embrace convenience. Unfortunately, convenient, commercial diets seem to play a major role in a growing number of canine illnesses.

Commercial Diets

Commercial diets are exactly that, those that can be commercially purchased at retail stores or veterinary clinics. Most Americans feed their dogs commercial foods and most veterinarians support that decision.

Under the heading of commercial dog food, there exist several different categories. The first will be referred to as supermarket dog food. These are the canned, semi-moist, and dry (kibble) foods that are available at supermarkets, grocery stores, and warehouses.

The next category includes prescription dog foods. These are only available through veterinary clinics. They are produced in both canned and dry formulas and are tailored toward specific problems, such as kidney disease, bowel inflammation, etc.

Additionally, there are some commercial diets that are advertised as "premium" food. Available as canned food and kibble, these diets typically contain more consistent ingredients from one batch to the next. They are available at large chain pet-supply stores, but never at grocery stores.

Finally, there are increasing numbers of natural or holistic pet foods. These are available in canned, kibble, and even frozen formulas. They can be found at holistic and high-end pet supply shops, holistic veterinary clinics, and over the Internet.

The Benefits of Feeding Commercial Pet Foods

Many veterinarians will recommend prescription or premium dog foods for their patients. This may include an ever-growing selection of high-fiber, low-fat, and low-protein formulations geared toward such conditions as obesity, inflammatory bowel disease, skin allergies, and kidney degeneration. Different veterinarians have their personal favorites, as do dogs and their owners. Commercial diets are convenient for the dog owner. Dispensing a measured amount keeps mealtime uncomplicated.

Those are the benefits to feeding commercial food. As more literature becomes available regarding the role of diet in healthcare, however, it is valuable to examine the content and effects of commercial diets. Following are a number of interesting findings. Some of them are newly published; others have been around for some time.

The Drawbacks of Feeding Commercial Pet Foods

To best understand this discussion, it is important to examine the physical design of the dog and what food is most appropriate for him. Some people believe that domestic dogs have adapted, anatomically, to their environment. They believe that over time the dog's digestive system has radically changed from that of his ancestor, the wolf. Most canine nutritionists disagree. They support the concept that dogs still maintain the inner workings of the wolf. Since there is much evidence to support this concept, let us begin here and consider the diet of the wild dog or wolf.

Paleontologists estimate that a period of approximately 100,000 years is required before evolutionary changes occur within a species. The most accepted theories estimate that dogs began their association with humans between 10,000 and 15,000 years ago. This is a much shorter time span than that considered necessary for evolutionary changes.

Dogs and wolves are physically very similar. Their DNA differs by only 1% to 2%. Humans have certainly manipulated the superficial appearance of the dog through selective breeding, but have not altered the dog's basic digestive workings at all.

Dogs and wolves are *primarily* designed to eat meat. They may scavenge many things, but their anatomy reveals much about which foods are, and are not, appropriate for them. Examine their teeth and jaws. They are designed for grasping and tearing meat. Dogs quickly gulp their food. This is quite different from herbivores and some omnivores that have broad, flat teeth designed for leisurely chewing.

As another comparison, human saliva contains amylase, an enzyme that aids in digestion. Amylase begins to break down carbohydrates during mastication (chewing). No digestive enzymes are present in the dog's saliva. Canine digestion does not begin until food reaches the stomach.

In addition to being a meat eater, the dog is also a scavenger. If something smells edible to him, and he is given the opportunity, a dog will eat almost anything. This includes decaying carcasses and animal droppings.

Depending on locale, a springtime diet of the wolf may include the eggs of waterfowl, young hatchlings, fish, and small birds. Summertime may bring a diet of rodents, pheasant, wild turkey, green vegetation, and fallen fruit. In autumn, many of today's wolves find injured deer or piles of innards left behind by human hunters. Large prey is frequently hidden or buried to be finished at a later time. Winter is a fight for whatever can be found.

Dogs are physically and metabolically designed to eat these foods. They possess very **strong stomach acids** and **short digestive tracts**. Many nutritionists believe that, together, these protect the dog from numerous and ever-present germs in his environment. (Remember: Dogs frequently eat and roll in feces and decayed carcasses as part of their normal behavior.) Bacteria are either killed in the stomach or hastened through the system before they can have any effect on the animal. The dog was designed to digest his meal *rapidly*.

With that history in mind, it is interesting to note how radically a typical commercial diet disagrees with the canine design. The topic of protein is as a good a place as any to begin this discussion.

Protein Sources in Commercial Foods

Most dog owners consider the term protein to mean meat. Grains also supply protein in the diet and they will be discussed in a later section. Here, we will examine meat and its by-products.

In most commercial dog food, the meats being used have been declared "unfit for human consumption." Occasionally, it is possible to find a commercial pet food that contains high-quality, human-grade meat, but this is rare and proudly advertised when it is the case. The meats found in most commercial dog food are, in essence, **the waste products** of the slaughterhouse industry. They are euphemistically referred to as the "4-Ds," livestock that is diseased, disabled, dead, or in the process of dying on the way to slaughter.

Meat by-products, meat by-product-meal, and bone meal are other phrases that disguise non-nutritious waste products. Meat rendering plants that produce these products may use any of the following ingredients in the rendering process:

> Diseased companion animals euthanized at veterinary clinics and shelters
> Road-kill animals
> Zoo animals dead from cancer and infection
> Restaurant grease and garbage
> Supermarket meats long past their expiration dates
> Cancerous tissue and tumors cut away from carcasses

Cooking at High Temperatures

These ingredients are cooked at high heats (greater than 170 degrees F). This accomplishes several things. It helps preserve the food by destroying certain natural chemicals in the meat called enzymes. It permanently alters the arrangement of amino acids, the basic building blocks of protein. And it destroys a number of vitamins and essential fatty acids.

Enzymes

There have been about 4,000 enzymes identified throughout nature. They fall into three major classes: Metabolic enzymes, digestive enzymes, and food enzymes. All three are designed to work together in a beautifully balanced system.

Metabolic enzymes are present in the blood, tissues, and organs of the body. For example, white blood cells carry protease, the enzyme that digests protein. This enzyme is released against invading organisms as part of the immune system response.

Other examples of metabolic enzymes include liver enzymes and cardiac enzymes. These enzymes are responsible for cell growth and repair in their respective organs. Damage to the liver or heart can result in a release of enzymes into the bloodstream. You may have heard your own doctor or veterinarian discuss "elevated cardiac enzymes" or "elevated liver enzymes," such as alkaline phosphatase.

Digestive enzymes are those that the body produces to break down food into useable nutrients. In the canine body, the stomach produces pepsin to digest protein. The exocrine portion of the pancreas produces protease (which also digests protein) as well as amylase (to digest carbohydrates) and lipase (to digest fats/lipids).

Finally, there are enzymes present in all fresh food. They contribute to the breakdown of food (fermentation) when it is not preserved by chemicals or cooking. Nature's great design makes these available so the pancreas does not have to provide all of the necessary enzymes alone. While a minor degree of controversy exists on this topic, several studies indicate that **food enzymes** will digest 5% to 75% of the food itself, without the help of the pancreas.

While some foods (starches) are made more digestible by cooking, most are not. High temperatures (usually 138 to 170 degrees F) *destroy the intrinsic enzymes in fresh foods, causing the pancreas to work harder.* Over a lifetime, the pancreas has trouble keeping pace with the continual demands of a processed diet. Eventually, it may be unable to produce a sufficient quantity of enzymes. This may help explain why diseases of the pancreas are often seen in older dogs.

When the pancreas can no longer produce the necessary volume of enzymes, the body calls upon *metabolic* enzymes to aid in digestion. These stores can be found in the liver, spleen, kidneys, heart, and lungs. Enzymes are routed from these organs, through the bloodstream, and into the intestines to help break down food. High levels of enzymes in the blood, particularly serum lipase, are a good indication that the pancreas is overworked and inflamed.

The body can also draw additional enzymes from the bloodstream itself. The white blood cells contain numerous enzymes, including protease. Usually, this is used to attack invading organisms (which are proteins), but it can be very successful in aiding digestion. Many dogs with digestive problems demonstrate high white-blood cell counts.

However, this backup mechanism does have a flaw. When white blood cells are occupied with the process of food digestion, they are distracted from their primary role of protecting the body. Their ability to fight invaders is compromised. Completely processed diets may contribute to chronic infection and infestation.

When the pancreas is overworked or irritated, it becomes inflamed. Ultimately, the tissues of the pancreas swell and obstruct the pancreatic duct. This causes digestive enzymes to accumulate within the pancreas. The high concentration of enzymes overwhelms the system that normally maintains them in their inactive state. As this protective system fails, enzymes become active while still in the pancreas. This is known as **pancreatitis**. Auto-digestion, pain, vomiting, or diarrhea may result.

Incidences of pancreatitis are constantly increasing. This suggests that dogs have *not* evolved to effectively digest a diet of highly processed foods. If dogs had evolved to this state, the pancreas would be capable of meeting the great demand for digestive enzymes. Clearly it has not.

Bioavailability and Altered Nutrients

Cooking at high temperatures for long periods also alters the arrangement of amino acids. The greater the degree of cooking, the greater the alteration in amino acids. They become increasingly indigestible. These altered amino acids may appear in such odd formations to the body, that it may not recognize them as food sources. Instead, the immune system may inadvertently respond to them *as if they were invaders.*

About half of the altered amino acids in commercial diets are unusable by the canine body. In humans, inadequate supplies of amino acids have been implicated in a host of ailments. This includes impaired central nervous system function, impaired endocrine system function, and impaired immune system function. The brain requires a constant supply of useable amino acids in order to synthesize brain chemicals. Without intact, easily digestible amino acids, the body may have difficulty making hormones, enzymes, and neurotransmitters.

Protein that contains altered amino acids, chemicals, cancer cells from 4-D livestock, and is devoid of intrinsic enzymes, is considered to be poor-quality protein. It is difficult for a dog to absorb and utilize such protein. Canine nutritionists describe these foods as having "poor bioavailability." Poorly digested protein results in an accumulation of serum phosphorus.

Many dogs eating commercial diets eventually experience some degree of kidney or liver disease. Since these organs filter waste products from the body, they are constantly at work when so many impurities are present in the diet. When the liver is ill, medications and hormones, such as estrogen and cortisol, build up in the body. Bilirubin accumulates and can cause **jaundice**.

The heavy burden and constant inflammation also reduce kidney function. Healthy kidney tissue is replaced by scar tissue that can no longer filter urine. This creates a vicious cycle of further scarring and greater loss of function. Waste products, such as **urea,** can accumulate in the body and contribute to seizures.

Consider, again, the diet of the wild dog. His diet consists of 50% to 70% meat and meaty bones. His body secretes protein-digesting enzymes in two locations. His brain requires phosphorus (a product of protein digestion) for cell membrane function (**phospho**lipids), and energy production via the ATP (adenosine tri**phosphate**) molecule. These facts support the belief that dogs are designed to eat a diet rich in protein. Yet, many dog owners are led to believe that commercial diets consisting of only 20% protein are *too rich* for their dogs.

This conflict exists because the statistics printed on pet food labels reflect only how a food breaks down *chemically*. This is not a reflection of the food's bioavailability, that is, whether the body can actually use it. In the final analysis, it is much more likely that *poor-quality* protein is responsible for kidney degeneration, rather than the *quantity* of protein.

Cooking at high temperatures also damages the bioavailability of other nutrients, such as Vitamin C, the B vitamins, and essential fatty acids: All of which are necessary for proper neural function. Typically, vitamin supplements are added back into batches of commercial food at the end of the production process. However, they are not necessarily as available to the body (easy to use) as they were in their original and more natural form.

The B vitamins are especially important to normal brain health. Adequate levels of B6 and the amino acid methionine contribute to the production of the calming neurotransmitter, GABA. When insufficient levels of either are present, GABA production suffers. Vitamin B6 is also responsible for converting **homocysteine**, a by-product of methylation, back to methionine. (See page 19.) If there are insufficient levels of the B vitamins or magnesium, homocysteine accumulates and becomes a powerful convulsant.

Slowed Digestion

Insufficient food enzymes and altered amino acids have a similar effect on the dog. The pancreas is called upon to increase the production and secretion of digestive enzymes. This takes time, and significantly slows the rate of digestion. In her article, "Anatomy of a Carnivore and Dietary Needs", Dr. Lew Olson explains that wild dogs and wolves digest their meals in a matter of four or six hours, while in contrast, it can take eight to 15 hours for commercial dog food to break down, clear the stomach, and pass through the small intestine.

During this extended period, chemicals and other impurities have ample time to irritate and inflame the intestinal wall. The canine GI system was not designed to handle this. It was designed to process food quickly. Prolonged digestion lays the groundwork for disaster.

Fiber in Commercial Foods

Peanut hulls, almond shells, empty grain hulls, and beet pulp can all be added to commercial food as fiber. Beet pulp is the dried residue of sugar beets, essentially just sugar, which places a high demand on the endocrine pancreas to constantly produce insulin. The hulls of nuts and grains are used as fillers. They are used in many "lite" or "diet" formulations of pet foods, constituting as much as 15% of the diet.

None of these elements are natural to the dog. And given a choice, a dog would probably not eat these things on his own. In fact, many dogs intelligently refuse to eat these diets. They may forage elsewhere (including gardens, garbage cans, and countertops) in an attempt to find the nutrients they crave.

Fats in Commercial Foods

Dietary fat is blamed for a host of problems in dogs, including pancreatitis. This idea warrants closer examination. Dogs *do* require a certain amount of fat in their diet, so it should not be considered as the all-evil ingredient. Fat supplies essential fatty acids crucial to normal nerve cell function. And contemporary literature suggests that dogs utilize dietary fat as a primary source of energy—fat that is of high *quality*.

Fats, like protein, used in commercial dog food are usually very poor quality. They can consist of restaurant grease (often rancid and deemed unfit-for-humans) or the tallow that rises from vats of 4-D meats at rendering plants.

Poor-quality fat is responsible for the particular (rarely pleasant) odor of pet food. It is sprayed on to most commercial kibble to entice a dog to eat it. Although some commercial pet foods advertise supplementation with essential fatty acids (EFAs), it is important to realize that EFAs are easily destroyed by processing, refining, high temperatures (cooking), and prolonged exposure to air.

Consider again that puppies cannot digest all solid food early on. A fair comparison might be how we slowly and carefully offer solid food to our own children. We do not sit them down to a holiday dinner in their infancy.

The type of fat in most commercial foods (rancid and heavily preserved) is especially difficult for puppies to digest. It is devoid of its natural enzyme, lipase. Without sufficient lipase, the pancreas must work very hard to digest it. This places one of the earliest stresses on the dog's system.

Poor-quality fat irritates a puppy's sensitive intestinal lining. This leads to destruction of the epithelial cells and permanent, life-long scarring of the intestinal wall. This can cause the dog difficulty in recycling bile salts later in life. When the body is unable to reabsorb bile, it accumulates in the small intestine. Dogs often rid themselves of accumulated bile by regurgitating it. Usually this occurs in the early hours of the morning, when the dog's stomach is empty.

Intestinal scarring and alterations in bile recycling cause difficulty in digesting food particles and absorbing nutrients. A variety of nutrients are transported into the body *only* via lipids. This includes essential fatty acids and fat-soluble vitamins, such as vitamin A, E, and D. Absorption of important trace minerals, such as magnesium, zinc, and selenium, is also impaired when the intestinal lining is damaged or inflamed. If these basic building blocks cannot make it into the body, the structures that require them will function at a deficit. Heading this list are the cells of the brain and nervous system.

Chemicals in Commercial Foods

In addition to cooking commercial pet food, manufacturers must add a variety of potent chemicals to preserve it. Some of these include **BHT, BHA,** and **ethoxyquin**. BHT and BHA are usually prohibited in human food as they are known to contribute to cancer. These two chemicals cause abnormal brain development in infant mice. Amazingly, some of the *leading* brands of prescription dog foods contain BHT and BHA.

Ethoxyquin is essentially a pesticide/herbicide. Various industry sources label it, "*Caution — Poison*" and "*Toxic By Ingestion*." It has been implicated in a number of autoimmune disorders and need only be listed on the dog food label if it was added at the production plant. Ethoxyquin can be added at the feed grain mill or the rendering plant and *never appear on the label.*

Inorganic and toxic dyes are added to commercial food. Red, yellow, and blue dyes turn the food from gray to a pleasing reddish-brown color. Pleasing, that is, to humans. Dogs do not perceive color well, and color is not an issue in their eating habits. While these chemicals may help the *owner* find the food appealing, they may contribute to serious illness in dogs.

Artificial colors are some of the most hazardous chemical mixtures added to foods. A large percentage of them have never been tested for adverse affects. Others are documented as toxic to the liver, carcinogenic to thyroid and glial cells, or linked to adrenal gland atrophy in dogs. Studies done on human children demonstrate increased hyperactivity, restlessness, aggressiveness, and excitability several hours after ingesting artificially colored food.

Commercial foods contain many other additives in addition to dyes and preservatives. According to the Animal Protection Institute, pet food companies are not required to list these chemicals on product labels. Binding agents are added to the food to create the shapes of burgers and kibble. Clay products may be added to produce consistent-looking stools. Other additives may include anti-caking agents, drying agents, texturizers, stabilizers, thickeners, and flavorings.

Flavor enhancers such as phenols are classified as **endocrine disruptors**. Researchers have found that phenols attach to brain cell receptors normally intended for hormones such as thyroid hormone. If the receptor site is occupied, the hormone cannot enter the cell and perform its job.

Monosodium glutamate (MSG) is another chemical commonly used in pet foods to improve flavor. It can be hidden behind a number of terms, including hydrolyzed protein, gelatin, yeast, malt, natural flavors, seasonings, soy sauce, whey protein, and meat by-products. The primary ingredient in MSG is glutamate, the excitatory form of glutamic acid. Glutamate can stimulate many different types of excitatory cell receptors, and can be *so* stimulating as to actually cause brain cell death.

Normally, when a brain cell fires, channels in the membrane open for just a fraction of a second. MSG, however, causes these channels to stay open much longer. During this time, excessive amounts of calcium enter the cell, causing severe damage or death.

Excess calcium stimulates a feedback loop, which triggers the release of the body's natural glutamate. This, in turn, allows even more calcium into the cell. The end result is a condition called **excitotoxicity**. The cells become so excited, that they become permanently damaged or even die.

In addition, intracellular calcium causes the release of a metabolic enzyme called phospholipase. Phospholipase breaks down the **phospholipids** that comprise the cell membrane. The result brings us back full circle. Nutrients, ions, hormones, and waste products have difficulty passing through the damaged and less-permeable cell membrane.

In his book *Excitotoxins*, Dr. Russell Blaylock explains that the damage caused by MSG is not limited to brain cells. MSG has also been shown to damage the retinal cells of mice. Experts believe that it damages the hypothalamus of developing animals, resulting in endocrine problems and miswiring, later in life. Animals fed MSG have higher than average levels of **cortisol** and lower than average levels of thyroid hormone.

To illustrate the harsh and indigestible nature of these chemicals, it is worth noting that many of these additives also have industrial uses. They are used in the production of fertilizers, cement and mortar mixtures, insecticides, explosives, and industrial cleaners. *Over the past few decades*, the level of chemicals found in most commercial food has increased. Epileptic-dog owners routinely report the reduction of seizure activity when foods containing these chemicals are removed from the diet.

Grains and the Endocrine Pancreas

Most commercial diets are not well suited to the dog's physical make up and metabolism. In other words, they are not "biologically appropriate." They are primarily comprised of grain products.

Contemporary canine nutritionists explain that dogs do not process *complex* carbohydrates (grains) well. Studies demonstrate that unlike humans, dogs do not "carbo-load." That is, they do not store up energy from meals high in complex carbohydrates. While human athletes successfully practice this technique, it results in an accumulation of lactic acid in dogs. (Lactic acid causes the muscular pain experienced after unaccustomed exercise.) This demonstrates a marked difference in how dogs process complex carbohydrates.

Dog food labels list ingredients by weight, not volume, so lightweight grains can constitute the bulk of the ingredients without appearing first on the list. These diets can contain as much as 65% corn, wheat, rice, oats, barley, soy, rye, or combinations or components, thereof.

As previously mentioned, the dog is not physically designed to process large amounts of grain. Some is usually tolerated and certain dogs can even live long lives subsisting on a mainstay of grain. However, the average dog does not.

The makers of premium and prescription dog foods advertise the use of high-quality, whole grains in their food. They say these provide an "excellent source of protein" for dogs. Large amounts of grain may be an appropriate source of protein for some species, but *not so* for animals primarily designed to eat meat. In fact, it is whole grains that contain **phytic acid**, a substance that binds with minerals — such as calcium, magnesium, zinc, and selenium — rendering them unavailable to the body. These minerals are important nutrients for normal brain health.

In addition, the scientific community is focusing on the relationship between **grain intolerance** (celiac disease) and a number of other diseases. Grain intolerance results in inflammation of the intestinal lining. Symptoms include abdominal gas, diarrhea, hypoglycemia, and malabsorption.

The least-tolerated of the grains are wheat, barley, and rye. (One of the amino acids found in wheat is actually the excitatory amino acid, glutamate.) In humans, there is a higher incidence of grain intolerance in epileptics, autoimmune thyroid patients, lupus patients, and Type 1 diabetics. There appears to be a genetic tendency involved with celiac disease. There is also some evidence that these patients develop related diseases if grain is not removed from the diet.

When whole grain *is* used in commercial pet food, it has often been deemed unfit for human consumption due to mold, contaminants, or poor handling practices. Some brands reportedly contain damaged, spilled, and spoiled grain known as "the tail of the mill." This can include the hulls, chaff, straw, dust, dirt, and sand swept from the mill floor at the end of each week.

Canine teeth are designed for tearing and ripping, not grinding. Unlike some other animals, dogs' saliva contains no amylase, the enzyme to digest carbohydrates. This places an added burden on the pancreas to produce enzymes. Grains are heavily used in dog food, not because they are *beneficial* to dogs, but because they are economical and readily available fillers.

Over the past few decades, the proportion of grain in commercial food *has increased*. A number of veterinarians and canine nutritionists are now beginning to question the heavy inclusion of grain in the canine diet, especially when fed to young puppies. Experts are implicating grain in an increasing number of **autoimmune diseases** being diagnosed today. Since the brain and immune system are inextricably connected, high grain diets may, indeed, have an effect on seizure activity. A review of the immune system will help explain why.

Part II:
Immune System & Endocrine (hormone) Function

A Review of the Immune System

The body protects itself from infection with an intricate system of endocrine glands, hormones, and cells. This is clearly evident in the intestinal tract. The "mucosal barrier" — a system that includes a mucous layer, tightly packed epithelial (surface) cells, and antibodies — normally prohibits invaders from entering the body.

When an invading organism (a virus, for example) enters the body, white blood cells respond by producing materials called antibodies. Antibodies read and remember the protein make up of the invader. They become programmed to attack that invader any time it is encountered in the future. This is the principle upon which vaccines are based.

One important family of antibodies is the immunoglobulins. Named with letters of the alphabet, each immunoglobulin has a different role in the immune response. **Immunoglobulin A** (or IgA) is secreted in a thin, protective layer in the body's mucous membranes. It is found in body fluids, such as tears and saliva, as well as in the lungs, urinary bladder, and the intestines.

IgA is considered to be the body's first line of defense. Like a row of soldiers, IgA prevents invaders from reaching the intestinal wall. IgA binds the invaders and removes them from the area.

During normal digestion, protein is broken down into short chains of amino acids. The body recognizes these *short* chains or simple protein molecules as food sources (friends), not invaders. These fragments are allowed to pass by the IgA antibodies and into the intestinal wall to provide nutrition and eventually form hormones and neurotransmitters. The body generally recognizes larger, more complex protein molecules as invaders (foes). Normally, these molecules are recognized and removed by IgA antibodies.

In some instances, however, large, complex proteins *are* able to infiltrate the intestinal wall. They slip past the IgA antibodies and then squeeze between the epithelial (surface) cells of the intestine. This occurs when the epithelial cells are damaged and when IgA production is insufficient.

The first example is seen in young puppies, weaned from mother's milk as early as six weeks. The intestinal wall of puppies is highly permeable at this age. Since puppies are commonly switched to a commercial food high in cereal (grain) content, undigested grain protein enters the dog's system early on.

In contrast, consider again, the wild dog. Pups in the wild still nurse from their mother, on and off, until about three months of age. Until that time, their immature bodies are not able or ready to digest all forms of solid food. This is a very different scenario than that faced by domesticated puppies.

The second example of infiltration may simply be a continuation of the damage begun in puppyhood. Some adult dogs exhibit problems with IgA production. The body either produces *excess* amounts of IgA or *insufficient* amounts of IgA. In cases of excessive IgA production, an overkill effect takes place. The antibodies begin to attack anything around them, including the healthy tissue of the intestine. In cases of insufficient IgA production, antibodies are unable to completely line the intestinal wall. Gaps exist between them. This condition is referred to as **IgA deficiency.**

In either case, large, complex protein molecules are able to pass through these new spaces. This may include: Meat proteins, altered by high heat and difficult for the body to break apart, or grain proteins, which the canine body is poorly-designed to digest. Since grain is the major ingredient in commercial foods, it is statistically likely that grain protein crosses the intestinal wall most often.

When infiltration occurs, the body reacts to these large protein molecules as if they are invaders, not food sources. The second line of defense is deployed. **IgG** and **IgM** antibodies infiltrate the area. These antibodies attack and destroy the large protein molecules just as if the protein were a viral infection. **IgE** antibodies cause the release of **histamine**, a natural chemical in the body, which is also designed to fight invaders.

Histamine is responsible for the signs we see in **allergic reactions**. Some veterinarians have noticed a link between allergies and seizure activity. Scientists suspect histamine plays a role in neuronal excitability and seizure susceptibility. If histamine targets the skin tissue, the result is itchiness, swelling, and rash. If it targets the GI tract, signs can include swelling, irritation, vomiting, and diarrhea. This condition is often referred to as **inflammatory bowel disease**.

Dogs with this condition may exhibit episodes of frantic behavior. They may slobber, lick their lips, or eat household items (such as pillows or carpeting) in an attempt to soothe their irritation. Chronic inflammation of the bowel can impair absorption of prescription medications and necessary nutrients. In addition, chronic inflammation allows the toxic chemicals present in commercial food to reach the liver via the common bile duct. Related conditions include colitis and malabsorption diseases.

In cases where the immune system is responding to dietary irritants and invaders, the lymph system is heavily engaged in the production of white blood cells. As a result, the absorption of fatty acids, usually handled by the lymph system, is interrupted. This also contributes to poor digestion of dietary lipids.

Cortisol — The Stress Hormone

The immune system responds to this systemic inflammation by releasing cortisol, a hormone produced by the adrenal glands. Cortisol is released in response to both psychological and physical stressors. This can include such events as home remodeling, loud noises (fireworks, thunder), visitors, the arrival of a new puppy, separation anxiety, or a trip to the veterinarian's office. Cortisol is also released in response to physical stressors such as vaccinations, surgical procedures, or large dietary proteins that leak through the intestinal wall. It is interesting to note that many epileptic-dog owners report a rise in seizure activity following a stressful event.

Normally, the body will shut off cortisol production once the stressor (inflammation) stops. In healthy dogs, this occurs when the hypothalamus recognizes that sufficient levels of cortisol are present and curtails the release of ACTH. This, in turn, shuts off cortisol production. Normally, it is a finely tuned system. However, if inflammation persists over time, the feedback system becomes damaged and ineffective. High cortisol levels persist. Since cortisol touches nearly every, if not all, cells in the body, excess levels have myriad effects.

Stress, and the resulting cortisol, alters metabolism and intercellular functions in a number of ways. Excess levels of cortisol result in a dramatic rise in blood sugar levels (**hyperglycemia**) by releasing glucose stores held in the liver and other large muscles. When the brain senses a rise in blood sugar, the pancreas normally releases insulin, the hormone necessary to move glucose out of the bloodstream and into the cells.

Processed diets that are high in grain constantly stimulate insulin secretion. This over-stimulates the insulin receptors on the body's cells. They become numb to the effects of insulin. Consequently, less glucose moves into the cells. This is sometimes termed "insulin resistance."

With time, the pancreas may have difficulty keeping pace with demand for insulin. Like other endocrine glands, the pancreas may become exhausted. Chronic hyperglycemia can overwhelm the ability of the blood-brain barrier to transport sugar into the brain.

The combined result is that **glucose cannot move into the cells**. This is particularly detrimental for neurons, as they rely on glucose as their source of energy. Blood tests may indicate sufficient levels of glucose are present in the bloodstream, but they may not indicate whether glucose is being *moved into the cells*. If the cells cannot obtain nutrition, they cannot produce energy — energy necessary for normal production of chemicals and transport of ions. The result is called neuroendangerment, the condition in which cells become much less able to effectively handle insult or damage.

Excess cortisol breaks down muscle tissue (**catabolism**), causing **muscle weakness** and wasting. This can affect the dog's skeletal muscles with signs of fatigue, lethargy, or reduced coordination. Cortisol can also weaken other muscles, such as the bladder wall and sphincter muscles, causing urinary **incontinence** and dribbling. It can affect dental health by weakening ligaments in the gums. It can weaken the heart, causing cardiac irregularities, murmurs, and congestive **heart failure**. Such cardiac damage can reduce blood flow — and oxygen delivery — to the body's cells. This is known as **ischemia**, which contributes to seizures.

The break down of muscle tissue also releases several important amino acids into the bloodstream. Specifically this includes two **excitory amino acids**, glutamate and aspartate, which mobilize calcium into the neurons and lower the seizure threshold.

Excess cortisol also breaks down adipose tissue (body fat.) This is known as **lipolysis**. This action raises levels of **cholesterol** and **triglycerides** circulating in the bloodstream. Catabolism and lipolysis are the same processes that occur during periods of starvation. Believing this to be the case, the appetite center of the brain erroneously tells the dog to eat more. So, despite the fact that these dogs have sufficient levels of circulating blood sugar, some still feel hungry. This is known as **polyphagia** (excess hunger).

Dogs with high levels of cortisol are more susceptible to infection since excess cortisol **depresses the immune system**. This includes both the production and function of certain white blood cells. Pathogens reproduce more freely and attack the body. Skin, ear, and urinary tract infections are commonly seen in these dogs. These dogs are less capable of fighting off infestation from worms, fleas, and other **parasites**.

When the adrenal glands constantly release cortisol, they release several other hormones, as well. They release adrenaline (epinephrine), noradrenaline (norepinephrine), and aldosterone. These hormones are believed to contribute to **hypertension** (high blood pressure). Adrenal testosterone is also released. The body converts this to a form of estrogen called *adrenal* estrogen. This is different from the *ovarian* estrogen necessary for pregnancy, but still has many of the same effects.

Excess **estrogen** is commonly linked to increased seizure activity. (Brood bitches may experience seizures during pregnancy due to the high levels of circulating estrogen.) Excess estrogen (ovarian or adrenal) binds with thyroid hormone or the cell receptors meant for thyroid hormone. This results in hypothyroid symptoms. (Such cortisol-induced estrogen binding is a separate phenomenon from the most common cause of hypothyroidism, which is autoimmune disease. Autoimmune thyroid disease will be discussed in an upcoming section.) Certain thyroid tests performed on dogs with high cortisol may identify normal *levels* of thyroid, but such tests do not recognize that the hormone has been **rendered inactive**.

Studies indicate that high levels of cortisol also reduce the rate at which the stored-form of thyroid hormone (T4) is converted to active thyroid hormone (T3). If these dogs are only tested for levels of T4, the tests will not reflect the **interrupted conversion**.

Finally, high levels of ACTH are believed to **suppress the production of thyroid stimulating hormone (TSH)**, resulting in reduced levels of thyroid hormone. Consequently, when cortisol levels are high, thyroid levels may be low. (See Chapter 11, *Additional Health Concerns,* for details of thyroid testing and treatment.)

Cortisol increases the filtration rate of the kidneys, causing excessive urination (**polyuria**) and excessive drinking (**polydipsia**). Polyuria, in turn, results in excessive excretion of **magnesium** and **taurine**, one of the calming neurotransmitters. Polyuria also causes the retention of sodium molecules and a rise in blood pressure. When sodium levels outweigh potassium levels in the body, the sodium-potassium pump slows and calcium has a greater chance to enter neurons. This contributes to excess **neuromuscular excitability** and reduced seizure threshold.

Without magnesium, calcium cannot be deposited into skeletal bone. High levels of calcium remain circulating in the bloodstream and become deposited in soft tissue, instead.

Without magnesium, **homocysteine**, the end product of the methylation process, cannot be converted back to methionine, the harmless amino acid. Instead, homocysteine levels rise, becoming a powerful convulsant.

High-cortisol dogs commonly experience **heat intolerance.** These dogs pant excessively and may seek cool surfaces to dissipate their body heat. This problem can stem from several factors. First, excess cortisol raises the body temperature in an attempt to kill perceived invaders. Second, a scenario is created in which magnesium levels are deficient and cortisol levels are in excess. This results in **potassium** being moved out of the cells, into the bloodstream, and excreted by urination. (**Magnesium** normally maintains potassium *inside* the cells and sodium in the fluid *around* the cells.) Potassium loss results in symptoms of fatigue and heat exhaustion. Finally, high levels of cortisol damage the neurons in the hypothalamus and, in fact, damage neurons in many areas of the brain. As these cells die, vital functions, such as temperature control, may be lost.

Calcium and **phosphorus** levels are normally maintained at a 2:1 ratio in the body. When the body has difficulty breaking down and excreting poor-quality dietary protein, **phosphorus** accumulates. The body tries to maintain the normal ratio by raising levels of serum calcium. To achieve this, the body increases parathyroid gland activity (**hyperparathyroidism**) and secretes hyperparathyroid hormone. This activity pulls calcium from the intestinal tract, or from skeletal bones and cartilage. This is known as **demineralization**. This scenario may contribute to joint and bone pain (limping) and collapsed tracheal cartilage.

In these cases, calcium may also be deposited into the body's soft tissues. Such areas include the skin (resulting in itchy sores known as **calcinosis cutis**), the lungs, bladder (**calcium stones**), skeletal joints (resulting in signs of **arthritis**) and, some experts believe, the corneal and lens tissues of the eye. In human epileptics, there is evidence that calcium is also deposited in **brain** tissue, contributing to seizure activity.

Chronic excesses of cortisol cause lesions to develop on the liver. Such **liver disease** can raise levels of circulating liver enzymes such as alkaline phosphatase. Such damage may impair the liver's ability to break down chemicals, medications, and hormones.

Cortisol, along with excess calcium, breaks down **phospholipids** in neural cell membranes. This change in cell membranes drastically affects cell function. Altered membranes are more fragile and sensitive to attack. Researchers believe that nutrients, including oxygen and glucose, have greater difficulty entering the cell.

Excess cortisol has detrimental affects on cognitive function and memory, resulting in a condition sometimes described as canine cognitive disorder. Cortisol lowers levels of natural opioids and endorphins (the "feel good" chemicals in the brain) and GABA (the inihibitory neurotransmitter). The converse is also true. Higher levels of GABA lower circulating levels of cortisol. Signs of excess cortisol can include **mood changes** such as depression, aggression, stupor, hearing impairment, agitation, and confusion (circling and staring into corners), and seizures.

Related to nervous system function is that of ophthalmic function. Dogs with high levels of cortisol may experience eye problems including **uveitis** or **blindness**. This may include blindness related to hypoxia or Sudden Retinal Degeneration Syndrome (**SARD**).

Cortisol raises **platelet** counts. Circulating adrenalin increases the action (stickiness) of platelets. Together, they cause the **blood** to become thick, adhesive, and deliver oxygen less effectively. **Hypoxia** may cause seizures and transient blindness as it deprives brain and retinal cells of necessary oxygen supplies. (See Chapter 12, *Additional Health Concerns,* for more details on ophthalmic conditions.)

Patterns of Cortisol Release

Under normal conditions, cortisol levels follow seasonal, monthly, and circadian (24-hour) rhythms in humans and most other mammals. Levels are normally highest during the daytime and lowest at night. Cortisol has an inverse relationship with the hormone **melatonin**. Melatonin is produced by the **pineal gland**, deep within the brain, and is responsible for the waking and sleeping patterns of a normal circadian rhythm.

Melatonin levels are normally *lowest* during the daylight and highest as darkness falls. As levels increase, so does drowsiness. Excess cortisol disrupts this cycle. Many dogs may sleep during the day and experience varying degrees of **insomnia** during the night. Some dogs are **agitated** and **pace**. Others retire, only to wake their owners repeatedly during the night. Insufficient levels of magnesium can also contribute to increased irritability and insomnia.

Some sources identify lack of sleep as a trigger for seizures. Perhaps a more accurate observation would be that insomnia, magnesium loss, and seizure activity all have the same root cause. All may result from excess cortisol levels.

There is great importance to the natural ebb and flow of hormones. These cycles allow certain hormones to perform their jobs, while curbing the affects of others. This provides the body periods of rest. When cortisol levels are consistently high, however, the body gets no reprieve from the powerful effects of this hormone.

It is worth noting that a great many dogs **seize during the night**…a time when cortisol levels *should be* at their lowest but are not. Similarly, a number of owners are acutely aware that their dogs seize on a **monthly cycle**. Lunar, or monthly cycles, have been implicated in the occurrence of humans' seizures, for centuries. (In fact, it is this cycle that is responsible for the term "lunacy" — madness, which at one time meant convulsions.) In addition, some veterinarians notice an increase in new epilepsy cases during certain times of the year when cortisol levels rise even more. These patterns should not be ignored.

The High Cortisol Continuum

Chronic stress and cortisol release can push adrenal gland function into other, unhealthy patterns. The concept of **stress adaptation** is well-accepted phenomena. Biologists describe it as an organism's ability to successfully adjust to stressful changes in the environment. This process is marked by three stages: Adaptation, alarm, and exhaustion.

The first stage, **adaptation** is the period when one effectively manages a short-term irritant or stressor. *Chronic* irritation can lead to the **alarm phase** in which the adrenal and pituitary glands become enlarged from chronic demand. The feedback mechanism located in the hypothalamus, which normally shuts off cortisol secretion, becomes damaged. These dogs become "stuck in overdrive" and exhibit the signs of excess cortisol.

Chronic stress increases the chance that the body's defense mechanisms will be overwhelmed by disease. It is fairly well accepted in human medicine that when an organ is required to function excessively, degeneration usually follows. Add to this scenario a depressed immune system, a genetic predisposition, and known carcinogens in the diet, and you may have the perfect recipe for Cushing's disease: A tumor of the adrenal or pituitary glands.

Not all patients develop a tumor. Some individuals may pass from a period of excessive adrenal function to a period of excessively *low* function. This is the third stage of the stress response known as **adrenal exhaustion**. Classic symptoms include loss of appetite, lethargy, weakness, and depression. This scenario is also called **Addison's disease**.

Exhausted adrenal glands produce insufficient levels of cortisol, or cortisol that is biologically inactive. Inactive cortisol cannot perform its normal functions and does not register with the pituitary gland as "real" cortisol. Exhausted adrenal glands may no longer be able to respond to stress and may result in a "normal" **ACTH stimulation test**, which is used to measure adrenal function. While many practitioners take this to mean the adrenal glands are in good health, this is far from true. Dogs "stuck in overdrive", or the alarm phase, may also exhibit normal or only slightly elevated test results. This is due to the fact that although day-to-day cortisol levels are high, no tumor is present.

Part III: Genetics

Scientists explain that all the cells of an individual's body contain the very same DNA. Yet, cells vary greatly in their shapes, functions, and abilities. Just consider the different jobs performed by skin cells, blood cells, and brain cells, for example. How can these cells all contain the same DNA, yet function so differently?

Cells differ in their jobs and construction because minute portions of the DNA strand are turned on (activated) in some cells and turned off in other cells. Researchers believe that the process of methylation keeps the active DNA portions turned on and **the inactive portions turned off** throughout one's lifetime.

To review, methylation is the chemical process in which SAMe molecules donate a methyl group to carry out work in the body. If the body is unable to produce sufficient methylation due to free radical damage or lack of raw materials (magnesium, methionine, or ATP production), the cells may experience alterations. Active functions may be lost or previously inactive portions of DNA may begin functioning.

Scientists report that cortisol also interferes with the normal methylation process. Cortisol is capable of crossing the cell membrane without the need for receptor sites. Cortisol then binds with materials inside the cell and sparks a series of reactions. Ultimately, the portions of DNA that were once kept inactive are now "turned on."

As the cell reproduces itself, the altered DNA becomes evident in new and dysfunctional ways. The new function can be any one of a million things: The loss of an enzyme, the addition of a protein or enzyme, the inability to synthesize certain brain chemicals, or the growth of cancerous cells. This process is described as **gene transcription** or the **expression** of a genetic predisposition. Many illnesses, including idiopathic epilepsy, celiac disease, hypothyroidism, and other autoimmune diseases are considered to demonstrate genetic patterns.

Cortisol's Relationship to Autoimmune Disease

When the immune system is healthy, white blood cells are able to distinguish between friend (cells of the body) and foe (invaders). But when the immune system is highly stressed, it fails to make this distinction. Several factors contribute to autoimmune disease: A genetic predisposition, high levels of cortisol, and an offending protein.

As previously mentioned, veterinarians and scientists have identified that a genetic predisposition exists in a number of autoimmune diseases. These individuals and their family members are statistically more likely to develop autoimmune diseases.

When cortisol "turns on" the dormant portions of the dog's DNA, those cells in the body are reproduced in an altered form. Conceivably, the alteration could occur in the cell membrane. Proteins in the membrane normally indicate to the immune system that they "belong" — that they are part of the body. (See illustration on page 23.) If these proteins are altered in their amino acid make up, it's possible that they will no longer be recognized by the immune system as "self."

Antibodies that have been previously programmed to attack a foreign amino acid chain *recognize a similar chain* somewhere in the dog's own body. The immune system can no longer make the distinction between self and non-self. Antibodies attack healthy tissue. Following are just a few of the autoimmune conditions diagnosed in dogs today.

Addison's disease — the body attacks and destroys the adrenal glands
Autoimmune Diabetes Mellitus type I — the body attacks the pancreatic beta cells
Autoimmune hemolytic anemia — the body attacks red blood cells
Autoimmune hypoparathyroidism — the body attacks the parathyroid glands
Autoimmune thyroiditis — the body attacks the thyroid gland
Discoid Lupus — the body attacks the soft, connective tissue
Inflammatory Bowel Disease — the body attacks the large intestine
Keratoconjunctivitis Sicca (dry-eye syndrome) — the body attacks the tear glands

In humans we even see Antiphospholipid Antibody Syndrome — a syndrome in which the body attacks the phospholipids found in cell membranes and includes such symptoms as transient ischemia, heart valve disease, and epilepsy. Autoimmune diseases often accompany one another in genetically prone individuals. For example, type I diabetics frequently exhibit thyroiditis.

The connection between IgA deficiency, grain protein, and autoimmune disease is so well accepted in human healthcare that it has a nickname. It is called the "leaky gut syndrome." Studies indicate that humans with many of these conditions also demonstrate grain protein intolerance. *This includes epileptics.*

Thyroid Function, Metabolism, and Seizures

Hypothyroidism refers to the inability of the thyroid gland to produce sufficient thyroid hormone. A number of factors can reduce thyroid function. As previously discussed, excess cortisol (or prescription prednisone or other steroid-like medications) can suppress thyroid function.

Certain chemicals have been implicated in the disruption of hormone function. Chemicals found in commercial pet food, pesticides, herbicides, and some industrial cleaners bind with receptors on brain cells. Since these receptors are designed to actually receive thyroid hormone molecules, normal function is impossible. This is called endocrine disruption.

The primary cause of hypothyroidism in dogs, however, is **lymphocytic thyroiditis**, a condition in which white blood cells attack and destroy thyroid tissue. This is, perhaps, the most common autoimmune disease diagnosed in dogs. Like most other autoimmune diseases, there is likely a genetic component present in these cases, which may be triggered by an environmental factor.

Canned and processed foods often contain large amounts of salt. Today, salt is most often iodized (contains iodine). When significant amounts of iodine are consumed, it becomes concentrated in the thyroid gland as thyroglobulin (a hormone precursor). Some sources suggest that high levels of accumulated thyroglobulin initiate the autoimmune response.

Certain breeds seem more predisposed to thyroid disease. These include the Akita, Beagle, Boxer, Chow Chow, Cocker Spaniel, Clumber Spaniel, Doberman, English Setter, Golden Retriever, Irish Setter, Labrador Retriever, Miniature Schnauzer, Old English Sheepdog, Poodle, and Shetland Sheepdog. Of course, this list does not rule out the diagnosis of hypothyroidism in other breeds or mixed-breed dogs.

Thyroid hormone orchestrates the rate of activity and work in all cells of the body. A deficiency in thyroid hormone levels or activity can, therefore, affect a great many functions in the body. Certain signs of the disease may mimic those of high cortisol, including **lethargy**, **increased appetite**, **weight gain**, a **brittle coat**, or **hyperpigmentation** of the skin. Other signs can include increased **shedding** and cold intolerance (**heat-seeking** behaviors).

Studies in human healthcare have linked numerous **neurological alterations** with low thyroid function. Topping the list are depression, anxiety, and dementia. Some holistic veterinarians also link aggression and seizures to low thyroid function.

Thyroid hormone normally helps neurotransmitters attach to cell membranes. It also fuels the activity of the cell (metabolism, enzyme production, and the activity of the sodium-potassium pump.) When these processes are interrupted, alterations in **brain chemistry** result.

Low thyroid levels result in higher levels of certain white blood cells. This includes neutrophils, monocytes, and eosinophils. This can result in increased signs of **allergic reactions**.

Low thyroid levels are believed to contribute to **anemia**. This occurs because low thyroid function results in sluggish production of red blood cells and sluggish absorption of dietary iron. These two elements are necessary for the normal transportation of oxygen through the blood stream and into brain cells.

There are distinct connections between thyroid activity and adrenal activity. Certain **adrenal hormones** assist in the conversion of T4 to T3. Scientists believe that adrenal hormones influence the passage of thyroid hormone into the cells. Alterations in adrenal function — such as adrenal exhaustion or the production of biologically inactive hormones — are believed to affect thyroid function.

If a dog has passed from excessive adrenal function to adrenal exhaustion, further connections present themselves. If a hypothyroid patient is treated with thyroid replacement hormone, the rate of metabolism will rise. This increase can make the adrenal insufficiency more apparent. Signs of lethargy and weakness may remain; leading to the false assumption that thyroid treatment was in error. In human healthcare, these patients are treated with both thyroid and adrenal-replacement hormones.

Inactive or insufficient levels of thyroid hormone slow the rate of metabolism. If the cells cannot produce the energy necessary for normal production of neurochemicals and transport of ions, they become much less able to effectively handle any type of insult or damage. When energy is deficient, the brain cells are more easily excitable.

Part IV: Additional Environmental Factors

Chemicals, Pesticides, and Wormers

Increasing evidence suggests that environmental chemicals contribute to neurological, endocrine, and immune system dysfunction. Many chemicals break down into **free radical** molecules. They steal electrons from normal molecules in the body. This causes damage in various forms. Free radicals fuse the fatty acids in cell membranes, making them less permeable. They break off identification proteins in cell membranes and damage cells of the immune system, both of which may contribute to autoimmune disease. Free radicals damage cell nuclei, disrupting the DNA material found there.

It is common practice to use powerful pesticides on or near our pets. Some, such as flea bombs, carpet powders, weed killers, and garden pesticides, saturate the dog's environment. We place others directly on our pets: Flea collars, shampoos, and drop-on repellents that are so potent they persist for many months. And some, such as heartworm medications, we give our pets internally. Keep in mind that the product labels instruct *humans* to wear gloves and wash their hands thoroughly after contact with these chemicals.

Phenols are a class of industrial chemicals used as a flavor enhancer in pet foods and found in aromatic cedar products and pine cleaners. Phenols, as well as a number of yard and garden herbicides and insecticides, are classified as **endocrine disrupters**. Researchers have found that phenols attach to brain cells instead of appropriate hormones such as thyroid hormone.

The federal Environmental Protection Agency (FDA) has identified roughly 140 pesticides as **neurotoxins**. Included in this classification are a number of the chemicals commonly used to kill fleas, ticks, and heartworms. These chemicals act upon the brains of pests in order to kill them. Some chemicals act on the nervous system of mammals in exactly the same way they act upon insects. They interfere with biochemical brain activity, resulting in hyperexcitability and seizures.

Pet owners believe these preparations must be safe if they are sold in grocery stores or recommended by veterinary professionals. The law that regulates pesticide use — the Federal Insecticide, Fungicide, and Rodenticide Act — does not use safety as the measure for allowing a pesticide on the market. Instead, a risk-benefit standard is used. If the pesticide has potential benefits, it may be approved for use regardless of the hazards.

It is both fascinating and disturbing to note the relationship between pesticides and **kindling**, the phenomenon in which the brain's electrical pathways become increasingly established with each seizure. The more developed the pathways, the greater the likelihood that seizures will recur. Laboratory animals *are exposed to low-level pesticides in order to test and initiate the kindling response.* Many pesticides, including pyrethroids, inhibit GABA receptors and lower the seizure threshold. Exposure to repeated stress, such as pesticides, plays a relevant role in seizure activity. (See Chapter 11, *Additional Health Concerns*, for more natural methods of pest control.)

While not truly chemicals, a certain number of strong fragrances can precipitate seizures in dogs. Included in this list are fragrant **essential oils** used in aromatherapy, such as rosemary, sage, and pine. These oils are highly concentrated. They may be as much as *70 times stronger* than the actual herb, and consequently, may have a more potent affect on the animal than the actual herb. So, whereas an individual might have a seizure triggered by the *aroma of an essential oil,* an individual may have no problem from contact with the same herb in the diet.

Look around your house and examine your daily routines. Are there other house and garden chemicals that can be reduced or eliminated? Try to minimize the general load of chemical insults: Fabric softeners, dryer sheets, floor polishes, air fresheners, carpet-cleaner powders, spray on/brush out pet shampoos, insect repellant, weed killers, and furniture stain repellants. Living a more chemical-free life is beneficial for both you and your pets.

Vaccines

For years, the accepted practice has been to inoculate pets on an annual basis. This repeatedly and unnecessarily provokes the immune response, which includes cortisol release. Presently, veterinarians are departing from this philosophy. If you have an adult pet — older than three or four years of age — it is likely that he has developed lifelong immunity to the diseases for which he's been inoculated.

Many veterinarians now recommend against vaccinating a dog that suffers from immune-related disease. Dogs with compromised immune function may have an altered response to repeat immunization. They may develop encephalitis or meningitis, **inflammatory conditions** that have been linked to seizures.

In addition to cortisol release and its effects on the nervous system, vaccines deliver a number of other chemicals to the body. According to the Centers for Disease Control (CDC), the following are just a few of the filler materials found in vaccines:

> Mercury (thimerisol), a heavy metal known for its damaging affects to neurotransmitters, enzymes, and pituitary function
> MSG, a source of the excitatory neurotransmitter glutamate
> Phenols, which block the ability of thyroid hormone to appropriately interact with brain cells
> Formalin or formaldehyde, both classified as potent neurotoxins

The link between vaccines, cortisol release, and seizure activity is frequently demonstrated. There have been numerous reports of dogs' first seizures following annual vaccinations. Vaccine boosters have also reportedly sent otherwise controlled epileptics into status epilepticus.

Additional Environmental Triggers

Occasionally, a dog's seizures will be triggered by rhythmic noises or visual stimuli. Dog owners report examples such as flashing lights (Christmas tree lights), the sound of a vacuum cleaner, or rain pounding on the roof. Of course, it is possible that these dogs experience some degree of concomitant stress with the advent of housecleaning, holiday visitors, or rainstorms. Psychological stress can contribute to seizures and this will be more fully examined in Chapter 11, *Additional Concerns*.

Part V: Summary

Consider the rather vicious cycle we have just discussed: Puppies experience intestinal scarring and protein infiltration when weaned onto commercial food at an early age.

A highly processed, commercial diet subjects the body to:
- altered forms of amino acids and other damaged nutrients
- a chronic need for pancreatic digestive enzymes
- intestinal inflammation

Essential fatty acids and fat-soluble vitamins and minerals are poorly absorbed. Neuron membranes become less permeable.

White blood cells bring additional enzymes to supplement digestion, neglecting their job to protect the body from invaders.

Digestion is slowed.

Slowed digestion allows ample time for harsh chemicals and foreign molecules to irritate the pancreas, liver, and intestinal lining.

Constant inflammation of internal organs, as well as repeated stimulation of the immune response (vaccines and chemical insults) results in a sustained production of cortisol.

Excess cortisol causes the following:

- It breaks down body muscle into excitatory amino acids.
- It causes calcification of soft tissue, including brain tissue.
- It causes the blood to become sluggish, reducing oxygen flow.
- Cortisol increases insulin resistance, reducing the passage of glucose into cells.
- It causes excessive urination, magnesium deficiency and sodium retention: A scenario that permits excess calcium into the neuron, damaging cell membranes and causing neurotoxicity.
- Cortisol damages the liver, reducing its ability to filter wastes.
- It lowers levels of GABA and thyroid hormone while raising levels of estrogen.
- It is involved with genetic expression of hereditary diseases.
- It depresses the immune system, causing IgA deficiency, infection, and infestation.

IgA deficiency allows for the continued infiltration of complex protein molecules into the body.

IgG and IgM antibodies are deployed, which memorize the amino acid chains of the large protein molecules and attempt to destroy them. These antibodies later recognize that same amino acid chain elsewhere in the dog's body and destroy these tissues, too.

If thyroid gland tissue is attacked, thyroid hormone production becomes insufficient. If the cells cannot produce sufficient energy necessary for production of neurochemicals and ion transport, they become more easily excitable.

The addition of pesticides, phenols, MSG, dyes, preservatives, and vaccines, further interfere with endocrine function and normal metabolism.

The whole situation seems a bit like the chicken-and-the-egg puzzle. Dog owners want to know which of their dog's health problems initiated the others. In reality, these conditions are not *precipitated* by one another at all. These problems are simply different expressions of the *same root problem* — commercial pet food, excessive vaccination, and chemical exposure. The results include digestive disease, immune system failure, and problems of excess cortisol production or "the threefold effect."

Today, many dogs exhibit some degree of endocrine/digestive/immune disease. They suffer from skin infections, allergies, epilepsy, autoimmune disorders, vomiting, diarrhea, obesity, hypothyroidism, urinary tract infections, and incontinence. *Which particular* disorder they develop is likely a matter of genetic predisposition but, clearly, many of our pets are experiencing the same underlying problem.

Think of cortisol-related problems as a continuum. They develop over time and follow a gradual progression. During this time, the body repeatedly substitutes one metabolic function for another. In some respects, this is a credit to how well the body can continually adapt to physiological stress.

Older dogs may seem to experience multiple health problems or "fall apart" all at once. These problems occur simultaneously because the entire endocrine/digestive/immune complex is severely stressed. Since metabolic adaptations can progress for some time, owners may not realize the severity of the situation until the dog's entire system is taxed. So, while great pains are taken to classify diseases and their causes, it becomes increasingly clear that metabolism, hormonal activity, and even genetic predispositions are interconnected.

References

Belfield, W.O., "Idiopathic Epilepsy," *Your Animal's Health*, an online newsletter, www.belfield.com, January-February, 1998.

Berti, I., et al, "Usefulness of Screening Program for Celiac Disease in Autoimmune Thyroiditis," *Digestive Diseases and Sciences,* 45(2): February, 2000.

Blaylock, R.L., *Excitotoxins: The Taste That Kills*. Santa Fe: Health Press, 1994.

Bourre, J.M., *Brainfood: A Provocative Exploration of the Connection Between What You Eat and How You Think*. Boston: Little, Brown and Company, 1998.

Braund, K.G., (Ed.) "Neurotoxic Disorders," *Clinical Neurology In Small Animals*. New York: International Veterinary Information Service, 2001.

Carlson, D.G., and Giffin, J.M., *Dog Owner's Home Veterinary Handbook*. New York: Howell Book House, 1992.

Claudio, L., et al, "Testing Methods for Developmental Neurotoxicity of Environmental Chemicals," *Toxicology and Applied Pharmacology*, 164(1): April, 2000.

Councell, C., et al, "Coexistence of Celiac and Thyroid Disease," *Gut,* 35(6): June, 1994.

Dodds, W.J., "Autoimmune Thyroid Disease," *DogWorld,* 77(5): October, 1992.

Ganong, W.F., *Review of Medical Physiology*. Norwalk, CT: Appleton & Lange, 1993.

Gobbi, G., et al, "Celiac Disease, Epilepsy and Cerebral Calcifications," *Lancet,* 340(8817): August, 1992.

Goldstein, M., *The Nature of Animal Healing: The Path to Your Pet's Health, Happiness and Longevity*: New York: Alfred A Knopf, 1999.

Grabenstein, J.D., *Immuno Facts: Vaccines & Immunologic Drugs*. St. Louis: Facts & Comparisons, 1999.

Haessig, A., et al, "Stress-induced Suppression of the Cellular Immune Reactions: On the Neuroendocrine Control of the Immune System," *Medical Hypotheses*, 46(6): June, 1996.

Horger, B.A., and Roth, R.H., "Stress and Central Amino Acid System," *Neurobiological and Clinical Consequences of Stress: From Adaptation to PTSD*. Lippincott-Raven: Philadelphia, 1995.

Hughes, G.R.V., "The Antiphospholipid Syndrome: Ten Years On," *Lancet,* 342: August, 1993.

Kerr, D.I.B., et al., "Stress and Cortisol Modulation of GABA Receptors," *Stress & Anxiety*, (13): 1990.

Kubova, H., Folbergrova, J., and Mares, P., "Seizures Induced by Homocysteine in Rats During Ontogenesis," *Epilepsia*, 36(8): August, 1995.

Lendon, H., and Smith, M.D., *Feed Your Body Right: Understanding Your Individual Body Chemistry for Proper Nutrition Without Guesswork*. New York: Evans and Co. Inc., 1994.

Levin, C.D., *Dogs, Diet and Disease: An Owner's Guide to Diabetes Mellitus, Pancreatitis, Cushing's Disease, and More*. Oregon City: Lantern Publications, 2001.

Lombard, J., and Germano, C., *The Brain Wellness Plan*. New York: Kensington Publishing Corporation, 1998.

Magaudda, A., et al, "Bilateral Occipital Calcification, Epilepsy and Coeliac Disease: Clinical and Neuroimaging Features of a New Syndrome," *Journal of Neurology, Neurosurgery, and Psychiatry*, 56(8): August, 1993.

Mount Sinai Comprehensive Epilepsy Center staff, "Seizure Provoking Factors," http://epilepsy.med.nyu.edu/Book/provoke.html, October, 2001.

Natori, Y., et al, "Changes of Thyroid Hormone Levels During ACTH Therapy in Epileptic Children," *Rinsho Byori,* (article originally in Japanese) July, 1994.

Oliver, J.E., Lorenz, M.D., and Kornegay, J.N., *Handbook of Veterinary Neurology, Third Edition*. Philadelphia: WB Saunders Company, 1997.

Olson, L., "Anatomy of a Carnivore and Dietary Needs," *B-Natural's Newsletter,* Spring, 1999.

Osiecki, H., *The Physician's Handbook of Clinical Nutrition.* Kelvin Grove, Australia: Bio Concepts Publishing, 1995.

Raber, J., "Detrimental Effects of Chronic Hypothalamic-Pituitary-Adrenal Axis Activation," *Molecular Neurobiology*, August, 1998.

Richard, A., and Reiter, J., *Epilepsy: A New Approach.* New York: Prentice Hall, 1990.

Rosenberger, B., *Life Itself: Exploring the Realm of the Living Cell.* Oxford: Oxford Press, 1998.

Sapolsky, R.M., *Why Zebras Don't Get Ulcers: An Updated Guide to Stress, Stress Related Disease, and Coping.* New York: W.H. Freeman & Co., 1998.

Sarjeant, D., and Evans, K., *Hard to Swallow: The Truth About Food Additives.* Burnaby, BC: Alive Books, 1999.

Scott, D.W., Miller, W.H., and Griffin, C.E., *Muller & Kirk's Small Animal Dermatology.* Philadelphia: W.B. Saunders Co., 2000.

Shames, R., and Shames K.H., *Thyroid Power: Ten Steps to Total Health.* New York: Harper Resource, 2001.

Smith, J.B., and Cowchock, F.S., "Antiphospholipid Antibodies: Clinical and Laboratory Considerations, Pathophysiology, and Treatment," *Immunology and Allergy Clinics of North America,* 14(4): April, 1994.

Strombeck, D.R., *Home Prepared Dog & Cat Diets: The Healthful Alternative.* Ames: Iowa State University Press, 1999.

Tuomisto, L., et al, "Modifying Effects of Histamine on Circadian Rhythms and Neuronal Excitability." *Behavioral Brain Research,* 124(2): October, 2001.

Vliet, E.L., *Screaming to be Heard: Hormone Connections Women Suspect and Doctors Ignore.* New York: M. Evans and Company, Inc., 2001.

Wulff-Tilford, M.L., and Tilford, G.L., *Herbs for Pets.* Irvine: Bow Tie Press, 1999.

Chapter 6

Overview of Treatments

The remainder of this book will focus on ways to minimize your dog's seizure activity. Prescription medication is, by far, the most prevalent method of treatment. However, a multifaceted approach may reduce seizure activity even further. These modalities will be discussed more fully in the upcoming chapters.

Antiepileptic Drugs (AEDs)

AEDs are highly effective in preventing or reducing seizures but they do not address the underlying cause of the problem. The goal of medical treatment is to balance a reduction in seizures with the side effects of the medications. Fine-tuning takes time and may require individualized care plans.

Dietary

Countless dog owners report a reduction in seizure activity after changing the dog's diet. One example is switching from budget commercial food to a premium or holistic brand. Reportedly, dogs switched to homemade meals do even better. This includes both home-cooked and fresh food (raw) diets. Some owners report a significant drop in medication levels or the absence of seizures for many consecutive months.

Kokopelli Mrs. Emma Peel CGC was switched to a fresh food diet with excellent results.

Prior to dietary changes, Emma seized approximately once each week. In the first year following these changes Emma experienced only five seizures. Now, in her second year of a fresh food diet, Emma has remained seizure-free for 10 months.

Additionally, during this time Emma's AEDs have been reduced by 60% and thyroid supplements by 30%. Emma receives minimal vaccines.

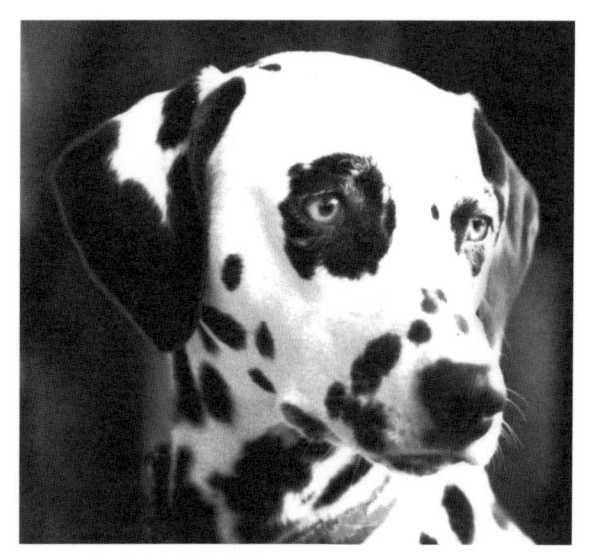

Photo courtesy of Marion Mitchell

Environmental

The dog owner is advised to minimize chemical irritants in his dog's environment. This includes chemicals used in the house, the yard, and those delivered directly to the dog.

Alternative Therapies

Acupuncture, chiropractic treatment, herbs, massage, and even exercise can be effective, ancillary forms of therapy. You may be able to perform some of these modalities at home with your dog. In other cases, it is best to secure the services of a qualified practitioner, specifically for acupuncture/Chinese medicine and chiropractic treatment. These are modalities of which Western medicine has long been critical but which are gaining increasing acceptance by dog owners.

Surgery

In a few situations, surgery may be indicated to reduce seizure activity. In hydrocephalus cases a ventriculoperitoneal shunt may be recommended to drain excess CSF from the ventricles of the brain to the peritoneal space in the abdomen. Unfortunately, this procedure is not 100% effective and not indicated for every dog. Your veterinarian may also recommend surgery to remove certain types of brain tumors.

Seizure-Arresting Techniques

In human healthcare, patients are taught methods of stopping a seizure just before it becomes full-blown. These techniques introduce scents, sounds, or touch to interrupt the brain's impending electrical discharge. There is value in this concept since the fewer seizures a dog has, the fewer he may likely have in the future.

Keeping Notes

Many epileptic-dog owners keep track of details in order to formulate a general picture of their dog's seizure activity. Keeping such a journal can be helpful in identifying patterns in seizure activity and triggers, or behaviors that alert to an oncoming seizure. With this information, it may be possible to reduce or minimize seizure activity.

Purchase a small notebook or a calendar that has enough space to make notes. Jot down any of the details you can remember from previous seizures, as well as all those that follow. Bring your seizure journal with you to veterinary appointments, both planned and emergency. Your notes may help you answer the veterinarian's questions during stressful moments or simply supply helpful details for future treatment.

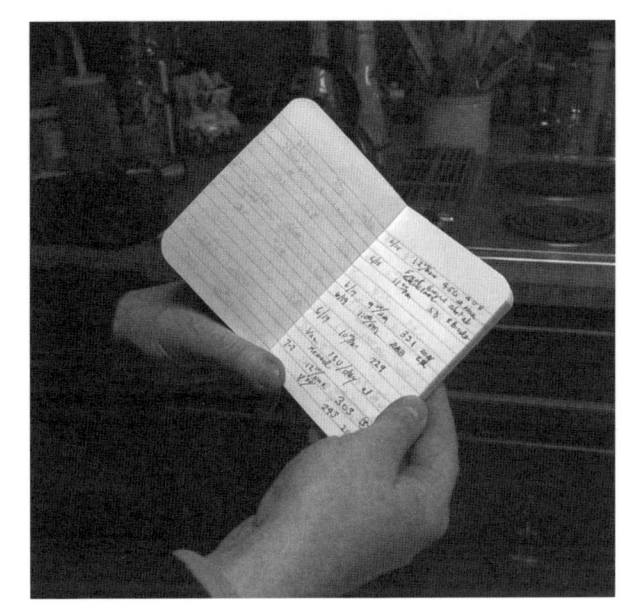

Include the following details in your notes:

> The time and date of the seizure
> The dog's location (room, car, public park, etc.) during the seizure
> What activities or incidents preceded the seizure (exercise, vacuuming, etc.)
> Pre-seizure behaviors (pacing, licking, unusual eye contact, and the length of time they began prior to the seizure)
> A description of the seizure (type, severity, loss of bladder control, length of duration, etc.)
> Post-seizure behaviors (type and duration)
> Include both the dog's behaviors and yours, such as medications or supplements you gave after the seizure and any arresting techniques that you believe successfully stopped or minimized the event

In addition, include:

> The dates that medication levels were changed and by what amount
> The dates of pesticide applications
> The results of laboratory tests

References

National Institute of Neurological Disorders: "Seizures and Epilepsy," http://www.ninds.nih.gov/health_and_medical/pbs/seizures_and_epilepsy_htr.htm, 2001.

Richard, A., and Reiter, J., *Epilepsy: A New Approach.* New York: Prentice Hall, 1990.

Chapter 7

Antiepileptic Drugs

The medications prescribed for epilepsy control are called anitepileptic drugs (AEDs) or anticonvulsants. Medicating epileptics is a highly effective treatment but it is also a balancing act between seizure control and the resulting side effects. These may include lowered blood counts, liver damage, and drowsiness, among other things. Individual dogs may respond to medications differently due to differences in metabolic rates.

There are two schools of thought when it comes to medicating seizure dogs. In the first, doctors typically prescribe medications early on. They believe that with each seizure, the electrical pathways become increasingly established: A phenomenon known as **kindling**. The more developed the pathways, the greater the likelihood that seizures will recur and the more difficult treatment may become.

In the second school of thought, doctors do not prescribe anticonvulsants until the frequency of seizures becomes more established. Once a pattern is established, and anticonvulsants are prescribed, it is easier to discern if the medications are indeed helpful in reducing seizure frequency.

Cluster seizures are a bit different. Veterinarians generally agree that these must be treated immediately. In fact, since cluster seizures can be more difficult to control, some veterinarians immediately prescribe more than one AED in combination and at higher than average doses. Status epilepticus, a continuous and life-threatening seizure, is an emergency situation and is discussed at the end of this chapter.

It is important to give your dog each and every dose of his seizure medications. Do not reduce or discontinue AEDs without your veterinarian's knowledge and supervision. Omitting or delaying a dose can increase the number and severity of seizures. If medications are suddenly discontinued, the brain can rebound with a massive electrical discharge, or even status epilepticus.

Drugs may be prescribed in combination with one another. Medicating epileptic dogs is often an ongoing process — a matter of fine-tuning the dosages, which may include raising one drug and lowering another. Combining medications may allow for lower individual dosages than when a single medication is prescribed. This is valuable since it may be possible to avoid severe side effects by keeping doses at a minimum.

The ranges for normal medication dosing are often described in milligrams (mg) per each kilogram (kg) of the dog's body weight. To convert pounds to kilograms, *divide* the dogs weight (pounds) by a factor of 2.2. To convert kilograms to pounds, *multiply* the kilograms by a factor of 2.2.

Some veterinarians consider reducing the dose of AEDs after a dog has been seizure-free for one to two years. Others are willing to try sooner. This is a gradual process, requiring several months' time and should be done under veterinary supervision. A number of dog owners have found that certain life-style changes, in addition to AEDs, can contribute to a low-seizure life.

Phenobarbital (Pb)

Action

Pb is a fairly effective medication in reducing epileptic seizures in dogs. Pb acts as a sedative and anticonvulsant. It is believed to increase the activity of GABA neurons, which inhibit electrical discharge. Phenobarbital is often effective almost immediately. The levels in the bloodstream become stable within about a week's time.

When Pb is first prescribed, or when the dose is increased, many dogs experience symptoms similar to those of excess cortisol since Pb does have **steroid-like effects**. Most commonly these include increased thirst (polydipsia), urination (polyuria), hunger (polyphagia), panting, pacing, or nighttime agitation. Some dogs experience sedation. This period of adjustment usually resolves itself within a week or two. At this time, your veterinarian may wish to measure blood levels of Pb.

Phenobarbital Dosages

Veterinarians typically prescribe Pb prior to other AEDs. However, it can be restrictive in its need for consistent dosing. With some dogs, it can be difficult to maintain blood levels at a concentration (a **therapeutic level**) that will control seizures.

Pb must be given at fairly exact times during the day. Altering the blood levels by even a small degree (or time delay) may result in a seizure. If you know you will be unable to dose your dog at the appropriate time, consider dosing him *earlier* in the day (versus delaying the dose.) Discuss this option with your veterinarian.

Some owners devise simple systems to remind them when to give the dog's medication. For example, one owner sets the alarm clock as soon as she arrives home from work. Many owners are instructed to give a forgotten dose as soon as they remember. Some veterinarians will have the dog skip the dose if the error is realized close to the time of the next scheduled dose.

Phenobarbital is dispensed as small, white tablets, measured in grains or milligrams, and, sometimes, in solution form. Veterinarians often prescribe Pb at a rate of 2 to 4 mg/kg every 12 hours. Sometimes a dog will be initially dosed at a higher rate, called a **loading dose**, which will then be reduced later.

After your dog has been on Pb for about two weeks (the loading period), your veterinarian will recommend measuring blood levels of Pb to ensure that the therapeutic levels are being maintained. Blood levels ranging between 14 to 40 micrograms (ug)/ml are considered acceptable. Once a therapeutic level has been reached, blood levels are typically measured every six months.

As each dose of Pb is absorbed into the body, blood levels of the drug will **peak**. As the day progresses, levels will drop until they hit their lowest point. This is termed the **valley** or the **trough**. At that point, the dog must have another dose. A few dogs that experience tremendous highs and lows in blood levels of the drug may require a third, daily dose. Some veterinarians prescribe morning doses that differ from evening doses. If a dog typically seizes at night, the veterinarian may prescribe an evening dose that is higher.

Some owners are instructed to give an extra dose of Pb to gain control over impending seizure activity or cluster seizures. Pills typically take effect in about an hour. Discuss this option with your veterinarian.

If your dog continues to experience significant weakness following an increase in dosage, discuss the matter with your veterinarian. Long-term weakness, lasting several months, may indicate a slightly excessive dose for a particular dog.

Side Effects of Phenobarbital

Liver damage is a common side effect of Pb, especially with long-term use. Such damage can include elevated liver enzymes (ASP or ALT) and loss of liver filtering function. Such liver dysfunction is **dose-dependant**, meaning that the degree of damage is related to the level of medication. Lower doses typically result in less liver damage.

It is important to provide periodic liver function testing, especially if dosages are increased over time. Your veterinarian may wish to monitor liver enzymes via blood tests every six months. He may also recommend a more specific liver function test, known as a bile acid test, be done every three to four months.

Bile acid tests evaluate the blood flow to the liver and other functions of the liver. Blood is first drawn after the dog has been fasted (gone without eating.) The dog is then fed and a blood sample is drawn again, two hours later. Bile acid does not usually escape from the portal system of blood vessels in a healthy dog. If significant liver damage is diagnosed, your dog will likely be removed from Pb and switched to a different medication such as potassium bromide.

In addition to the steroid-like effects listed above, phenobarbital, like cortisol, can interfere with **thyroid function** and alter certain components of a thyroid test. Specifically, this includes a decrease in free T4 and total serum T4 levels. Other values may remain normal. This illustrates the importance of performing a six-panel test.

Since each dog metabolizes drugs at different rates, individual care plans may be needed. While a general range for Pb dosing does exists, it is possible for some dogs to be overmedicated on "normal" doses. Signs of overdose include extreme lethargy, loss of coordination, stupor, and slowed breathing.

Potassium Bromide (KBr)

Action

Potassium bromide has been used to treat human epileptics since the 1800s. When phenobarbital became available, KBr fell out of vogue. However, KBr has been rediscovered recently, and certainly, it maintains an important place in the treatment of epileptic dogs.

Bromide is a salt with similar actions to those of chloride. Bromide, like chloride, is a negatively charged ion that passes through channels in the brain cell membrane. This causes the cell to become hyperpolarized (possessing a highly negative charge). In fact, since bromide is a slightly smaller molecule than chloride, it may even enter the cell more easily than chloride. The highly negative state produced prevents the cell from firing. In this way, KBr helps reduce seizure activity.

KBr takes longer to reach therapeutic levels but it is also less restrictive — in terms of dosing — than is phenobarbital. KBr can be given once or twice a day. It can be given in liquid form, which can be helpful when the dosage is being finely tuned.

Blood levels do not reach a steady level in the bloodstream until several months have passed. Doctors may check levels after a month and then recheck again after two months. However, it may take several months for the drug to reach therapeutic levels. The goal is to have blood levels between 1200 to 2000 micrograms (ug)/ml. Levels higher than this may result in toxicity, which can actually increase seizure activity.

KBr offers the great benefit of being broken down via the kidneys, rather than the liver. KBr does not have any known liver toxicity. This is extremely helpful to dogs suffering from liver failure.

Dietary chloride — including sodium chloride, or table salt — can interfere with the body's ability to absorb KBr and increase urinary excretion of KBr. In other words, higher levels of dietary chloride/salt will result in lower blood levels of KBr. This does not become an issue unless you are interested in switching your dog to a new diet. (See page 102, "Switching Diets.")

Potassium Bromide Dosages

A great many dogs are dosed with both KBr and Pb, especially in cases when seizures are difficult to control. In these cases, the phenobarbital is usually prescribed twice daily and the potassium bromide is dosed only once, usually at bedtime. As the KBr is added to the regime, it may be possible to reduce the levels of phenobarbital.

Some neurologists are returning to the use of KBr as the *primary* medication prescribed for epilepsy. In these cases, the usual dosage is 22 mg/kg every 12 hours. Your veterinarian may prescribe a more intense dose for the first few days. This loading dose may be prescribed in an attempt to reduce high seizure activity more quickly.

KBr is administered in either capsules or liquid form. Liquid may keep best, stored in the refrigerator.

Your veterinarian may wish to monitor blood levels of KBr two to three months after therapy has begun. He may also recommend measuring blood levels after any changes in dose have been made. Thereafter, most veterinarians will wish to measure KBr levels at six-month intervals.

Side Effects of Potassium Bromide

Side effect of KBr can include gastrointestinal (GI) upset, vomiting, and diarrhea. To minimize this, some owners divide the dose, giving half in the morning and half in the evening. Administering KBr with meals can also reduce GI upset.

Bromide (in KBr) may cause an increase in chloride readings on certain laboratory tests because tests cannot differentiate between the chemical make-up of bromide and chloride. Other side effects of KBr may include increased thirst (polydipsia) and increased urination (polyuria) as KBr is a salt. Some dogs experience reduced coordination.

Discuss these problems with your veterinarian. Such behaviors may indicate a slightly excessive dose for your particular dog. KBr toxicity (overdose) includes extreme muscle weakness, lethargy, stiffness, and sedation. In humans, KBr can cause acne and skin irritation.

Diazepam (or Valium)

Diazepam, in dogs, works as a short-acting anticonvulsant and is gaining increasing acceptance in seizure control. However, its use is limited to a special class of epilepsy. It is used to break the pattern of ongoing, generalized, cluster seizures. This can prevent the potential onset of status epilepticus and save the dog owner emotional grief and costly trips to the emergency veterinary clinic. Since dog owners and veterinarians typically discuss this as the "rectal Valium protocol," the remainder of this section will use the term Valium.

Forms of Diazapam/Valium

Valium is available in several different forms. Valium solution is most commonly recommended for rectal administration. It is dispensed in small brown glass bottles or syringes prefilled by a pharmacist. Oral Valium may also be prescribed for home administration. Oral Valium is dispensed in small white tablets measured milligrams.

Some dog owners have administered Valium suppositories during cluster seizures but they have found the absorption rate to be much slower than the Valium solution. Suppositories have another drawback. They may stimulate rectal reflexes more easily than the solution might. The rectal reflex may cause the dog to move his bowels and expel the suppository. Keep extra suppositories on hand in case of this scenario. Store them in the refrigerator, away from food.

Veterinarians must supply dog owners with Valium or write a prescription to be filled at a local pharmacy. Hospital pharmacies are more likely to have the **solution form** on hand. They may dispense a small, glass bottle with several empty syringes. Alternatively, they may dispense a pre-filled syringe containing the appropriate dose for your dog.

Valium solution is not frequently prescribed for humans, so a pharmacist may be somewhat confused as to what you are asking for. Pharmacists sometimes attempt to fill the Valium solution prescription with a syringe of Valium *gel*. You will notice this error since the price tag for a Valium gel (Diastat) syringe runs several hundred dollars!

Action

Valium is believed to enhance the action of GABA receptors and thereby improve the ability of chloride to enter the neuron. This action hyperpolarizes the cell and increases the seizure threshold (reduces seizures). The action of Valium is short-lived, however, so it is not recommended for daily seizure control.

Liquid Valium administered *rectally* has a reported onset of action between 5 and 15 minutes. Its antiseizure effects last approximately 30 to 60 minutes. *Oral* Valium has an onset of 30 to 40 minutes. Antiseizure effects of oral Valium last for an hour or two. Owners remark that the onset of Valium suppositories have an onset of 20 minutes or more.

Diazapam/Valium Dosages

For dogs taking phenobarbital, the protocol typically recommends a **rectal** Valium dose of 2 mg/kg. (For dogs *not* taking phenobarbital, the Valium dose is typically lower: 0.5 to 1 mg/kg.) These rates are higher than those normally prescribed intravenously but they are necessary to obtain sufficient blood levels via rectal absorption.

Some veterinarians also prescribe *oral* Valium as part of this protocol. Owners may be instructed to administer oral Valium, at a rate of 1 mg/kg, every one to two hours for the 24-hour period following the onset of the cluster. Discuss this option with your veterinarian.

Home Valium Procedure For Cluster Seizures

In his article on home treatment for cluster seizures, Dr. W.B. Thomas outlines the protocol recommended by the neurology service at the College of Veterinary Medicine, University of Tennessee. In this procedure, the dog owner is taught to administer rectal Valium at home, which can be especially helpful for dogs that experience multiple seizures with a 24-hour period.

Rectal administration is a relatively safe, fast, and effective method of delivery, especially during seizures. Dog owners are instructed to initiate the protocol when a second seizure occurs within 24 hours of an initial, generalized seizure. This protocol is not recommended for dogs that suffer more isolated seizures.

If you are sent home with a bottle of Valium, you will need to fill the syringe yourself. Some owners fill the syringe prior to the time it is actually needed. Bottles and pre-filled syringes should be stored at room temperature, and away from sunlight.

Valium solution is usually dispensed in small, 10 cc glass bottles. The top of the bottle is capped with a rubber stopper and is covered with a metal or plastic outer cap. This maintains the Valium's integrity during distribution and storage at the pharmacy. The outer cap is removed when you are ready to draw up the first injection.

Syringes consist of a barrel and a plunger. The barrel is marked off in dosage amounts measured in cubic centimeters (cc's) or milliliters (ml's). These terms are interchangeable. The plunger is the portion that expels the liquid. Needles, too, will have protective caps at both ends.

Chapter 7 — Antiepileptic Drugs

Preparing a Valium Syringe

Slide the plunger up and down the length of the barrel, several times. This will help ensure a smooth injection. Remove the protective cap that covers the hub (the back end) of the needle. Firmly twist the needle onto the tip of the syringe. Use a new, sterile needle each time. (It is important not to contaminate the Valium that remains in the bottle for the next use.)

Bottled medications, such as Valium, are prepared under vacuum pressure. As Valium is continually withdrawn from the bottle, the vacuum effect will increase. This makes it difficult to withdraw any more fluid. By injecting a small amount of air into the bottle prior to drawing out the Valium, you can counteract this effect. If this is done each time, the vacuum pressure will not increase.

Step 1: Steady the barrel of the syringe between 2 fingers

Step 2: Pull back plunger past the mark for your dog's dose

Draw back the plunger of the syringe until you reach the mark that indicates your dog's Valium dose.

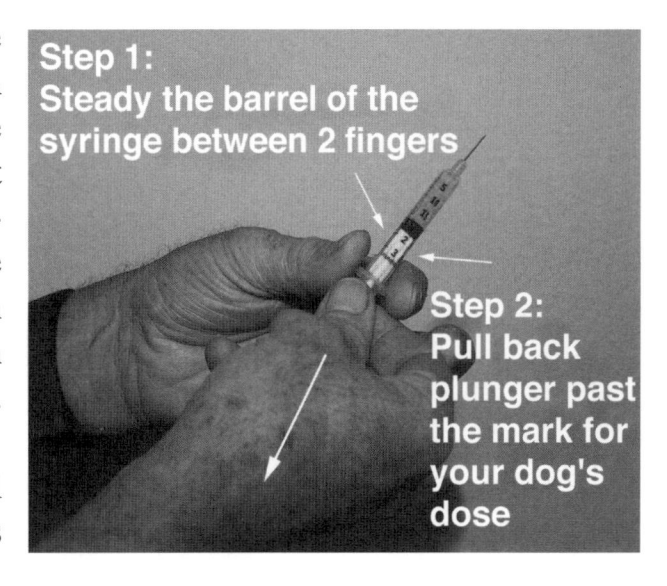

Step 3: Depress air from the syringe into the air pocket in the bottle

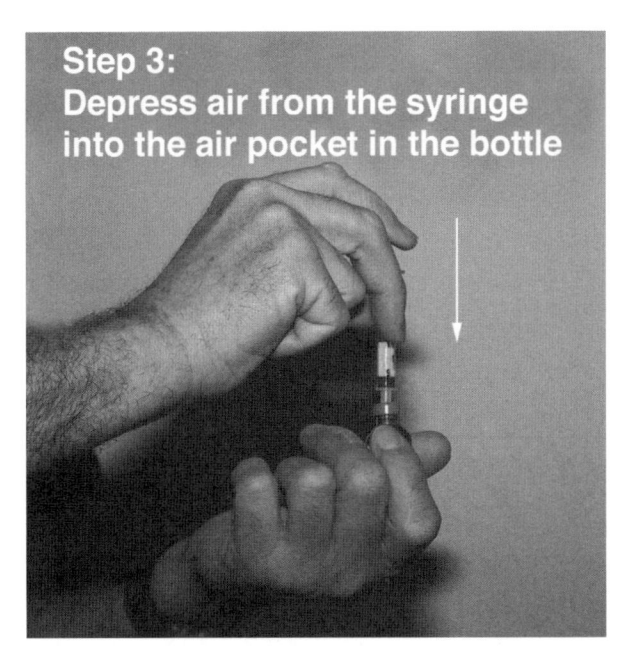

Flip off any protective caps from the Valium bottle. Insert the needle through the rubber stopper of the bottle and inject all of the air into the bottle.

Invert the bottle so the stopper points toward the floor. Slowly and gently pull back on the plunger. (You will likely have to hold the barrel of the syringe steady with your other fingers to keep the needle inside the bottle.) If you withdraw **only** air, pull the needle a bit further out of the bottle. (This indicates that Valium levels are low.)

Fill the syringe a little past your dog's prescribed dose. It is likely that a few tiny air bubbles will have entered the syringe and the extra Valium you have drawn up will be used to expel them. (Do this with the needle still inside the bottle.) Tap the syringe with

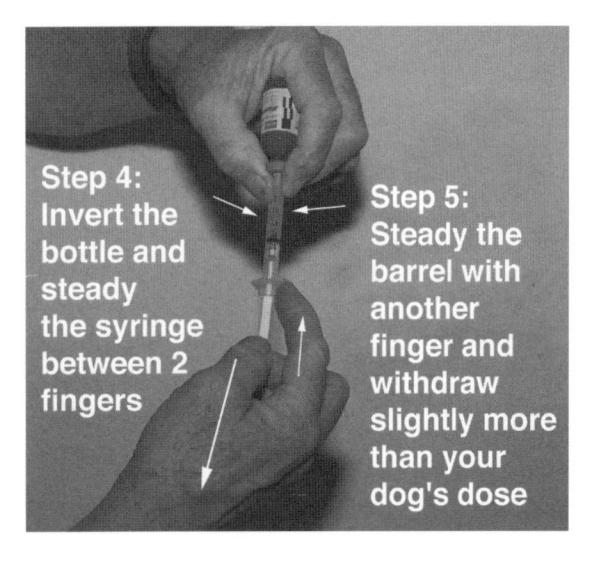

Step 4: Invert the bottle and steady the syringe between 2 fingers

Step 5: Steady the barrel with another finger and withdraw slightly more than your dog's dose

a flick from your forefinger. This should cause air bubbles to rise to the top of the syringe. Depress the syringe slightly, to expel the air bubbles back into the bottle. You should now have the correct dose of Valium for your dog.

Some owners use a magic marker to highlight the appropriate mark on all of their syringes, ahead of time. If you are simply preparing a syringe for future use, replace the cap on the needle and store in a cool (room temperature), dry location, away from direct sunlight.

Administering Rectal Valium

A **"Tom cat"-style catheter** is preferred, but a urinary catheter cut down to six inches will suffice. In the case of the latter, only insert approximately three inches into the rectum. Mark the appropriate distance with a permanent magic marker in advance.

Lubricate the catheter with a bit of KY, petroleum jelly or Vaseline. Once you have placed the catheter or your fingers near the dog's rectum, do not return to the jar of petroleum jelly without first washing your hands. You will contaminate it.

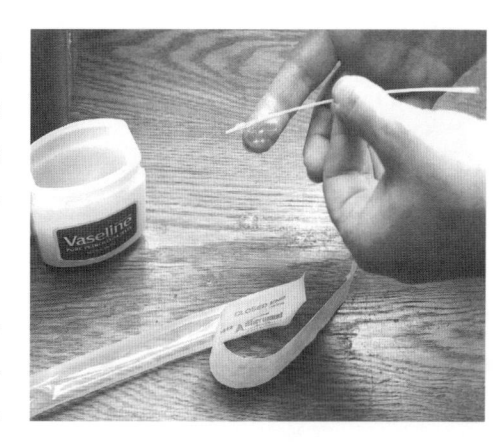

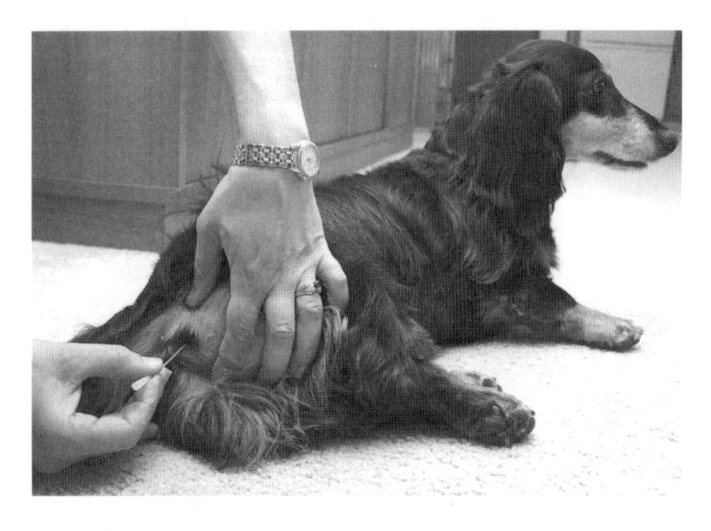

If your dog is becoming active and objects to your actions, ask another family member to gently restrain his head or use your elbow to block his head movement toward you. Most dogs are fairly groggy following a seizure, however, and have no interest in your activities.

Gently lift his tail and insert the catheter. Some owners insert the catheter, alone, and then attach the syringe *after* the catheter is inserted into the rectum. This allows any intestinal gas to escape before you attempt to inject.

Chapter 7 — Antiepileptic Drugs 85

Untwist the needle from the syringe and then twist the syringe onto the catheter. Be certain that the connection is tight or the pressure of the injection could cause the Valium to squirt out.

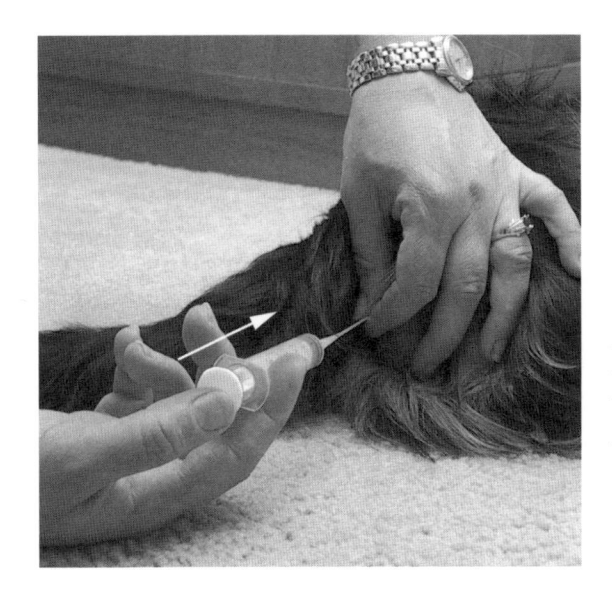

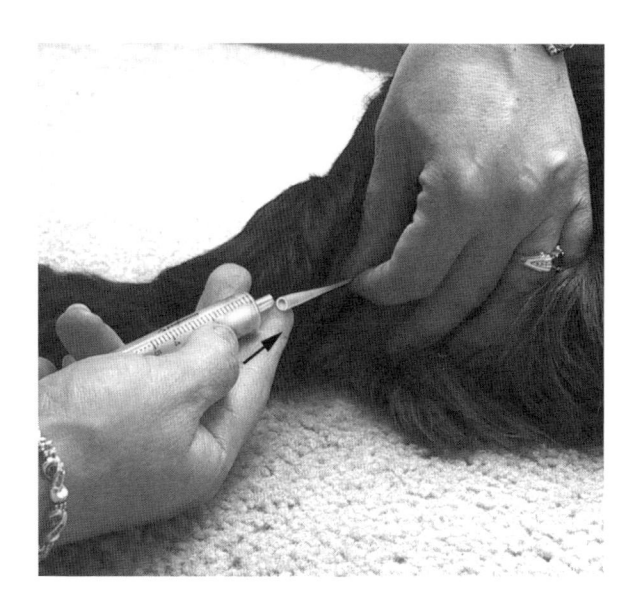

Hold the catheter and syringe horizontally, in line with the floor. This will aid in a smooth injection. Depress the plunger slowly and steadily.

Owners are often given the following instructions: **If seizures are not reduced in ten minutes**, the dose may be repeated once or twice more. If there is still no relief, owners should take the dog to an emergency veterinary clinic, immediately.

Do not attempt to clean and reuse syringes and catheters. Discard them after each use. Return needles to your veterinarian for appropriate disposal. Needles are considered medical waste and many areas have specific regulations regarding their disposal. If you obtain Valium bottles directly from your veterinarian, you may be instructed to return those as well.

If the thought of rectal injection intimidates you, consider practicing some of these skills before the onset of an actual cluster. When you receive your supplies, purchase a vial of saline, as well. You will be able to practice filling the syringe and getting a feel for how firmly to attach the catheter. If your dog is very mild mannered and obedient, and typically allows you to use a rectal thermometer, he may even allow you to practice inserting the catheter. If you wish to practice the latter, plan ahead by placing several food treats nearby so that you can reward him as soon as you are done.

If your dog is suffering from cluster seizures and his daily AEDs are not controlling them, you might wish to discuss this option with your veterinarian. (In addition, please consider some of the ancillary treatment methods discussed in the upcoming chapters.) Some veterinarians may be hesitant to prescribe a controlled substance such as Valium, for home use by their clients. They may worry that the drug will be abused. Dr. Thomas' article, as well as others, is included in the reference section at the end of this chapter.

If your veterinarian is still hesitant and alternate therapies prove unsuccessful, you may find it helpful to seek the assistance of a veterinary neurologist. These specialists are more familiar with the rectal Valium protocol and deal with it on a regular basis.

Side Effects (Valium)

Valium is not well tolerated by all dogs. Some owners report excitability, pacing, or whining, lasting for hours to days following administration. Others report that their dog is more disoriented than usual following the seizure. If your dog does not tolerate Valium, your veterinarian may be able to prescribe Clonazepam as a substitute. (See details below.) Many dog owners are instructed to reduce *oral* valium doses by 25% or 30% if their dog exhibits significant drowsiness.

In addition, there are some factors of *rectal* administration that are worthy of discussion. There may be fecal matter in the rectum. This may cause difficulty in administering the medication, or difficulty in how the body absorbs it. Rectal stimulation may cause the dog to defecate, as may the seizure, itself.

If the dog expels the Valium, or if Valium solution is difficult for you to secure, it is possible to simply crush Valium pills into a powder by using the back of a spoon. The powder can be mixed with a small amount of water, and dribbled onto the dog's gums or mouth. While absorption will be slower, this too should be absorbed across the mucous membranes. If your dog manifests snapping or aggressive behaviors, proceed with great care. Dog bites are painful.

Felbamate (or Felbatol)

Felbamate is prescribed for dogs that may be resistant to the previous medications. It is effective in 80% of cases but its action is unknown. It may cause liver damage. It is more expensive than other AEDs and must be given *every eight hours* at a rate of 15 mg/kg.

Clonazepam (or Klonopin, Rivotril)

Clonazepam may be used in dogs that cannot tolerate Valium. It is given every six to eight hours to ward off cluster seizures. If seizures are frequent, some owners are instructed to administer rectal Valium along with oral Clonazepam (instead of oral Valium).

Primidone (or Mysoline)

While this medication is approved for use specifically in canine epilepsy, it is losing popularity. Studies indicate that it is no more effective than other medications *and* it carries a greater risk of liver toxicity and irreversible liver damage. Most veterinarians will add KBr to the Pb regime, before they will add Primidone.

Medications Used in Status Epilepticus

Non-stop, or frequent cluster, seizures are considered an emergency situation requiring immediate care at the veterinary hospital. This may include intravenous drugs, such as Valium, phenobarbital, or *pento*barbital (a sedative that can provide the necessary time for phenobarbital to take effect). Your veterinarian may also supply intravenous (IV) glucose, electrolytes, or fluids.

Medication Refills

In general, it is important to refill AED prescriptions well before you finish a previous prescription. This is especially important for medications such as Pb, which must be maintained at consistent levels in the bloodstream, and Valium that is needed during more urgent moments. Once you bring home a refill prescription, calculate the days it will last. Make a note on your calendar as to when you should have it refilled. Remember that pharmacies occasionally delay orders and prescribing doctors may be out of town just when you need them. Plan ahead.

Prior to any trips you take, spend a bit of extra time to ensure that medication supplies will be adequate. If you are traveling *with* your dog, be certain that you have enough medications packed. Should you lose or damage your dog's pills it *may* be possible to have your hometown veterinarian phone or fax your dog's prescription to a local veterinarian. Be certain to take his phone number with you. Some owners also request a copy of their dog's medical record from the clinic. This can be valuable should your dog require emergency care at an unfamiliar clinic.

If you are boarding the dog, or enlisting the services of a house sitter, be certain to leave adequate medication supplies with the dog's caregiver. Leave written instructions as to how the medication should be given (dose, time of day, "with food," etc.) and what to do if a seizure occurs. Also, provide the phone number, name, and address of your regular veterinarian and any 24-hour, emergency clinics in the area.

References

Carson, J., "Treating Cluster Seizures with the Rectal and Oral Valium Protocol," www.canine-epilepsy-guardianangels.com, February, 2002.

Clemmons, R.M., "Seizure Disorders in Dogs and Cats," http://pawcare.com/rclemmons, January, 2002.

Kantrowitz L.B., et al, "Serum Total Thyroxin, Total Triiodothyronine, Free Thyroxin and Thyroxin and Thyrotropin Concentrations in Epileptic Dogs Treated with Anticonvulsants," *Journal of the American Veterinary Medical Association*, 214(12): June, 1999.

National Institute of Neurological Disorders: "Seizures and Epilepsy," http://www.ninds.nih.gov/health_and_medical/pbs/seizures_and_epilepsy_htr.htm, 2001.

Podell, M., "The Use of Diazepam per Rectum at Home for the Acute Management of Cluster Seizures in Dogs," *Journal of Veterinary Internal Medicine*, 9(2): 1995.

Richard, A., and Reiter, J., *Epilepsy: A New Approach.* New York: Prentice Hall, 1990.

Thomas, W.B., "Home Treatment with Rectal Diazepam for Cluster Seizures in Dogs," *Veterinary Clinics of North America: Small Animal Practice*, 30(1): January, 2000.

Chapter 8

Dietary Therapy

To most people, dog food means prepared food purchased commercially. This is a relatively new trend, however. Companion dogs have been eating processed foods for the just the last several decades. An ever-increasing number of medical researchers, psychiatrists, and veterinarians are realizing that a diet free of chemicals and mechanical degradation is an important therapy for disorders of both the mind and body.

A Review of Commercial Diets

As early as 1979, *Consumers Digest* questioned the logic of feeding highly processed, grain-based diets to pets. They reported, "There is mounting evidence that a lifetime of eating commercial pet foods can shorten your pet's life, make him fatter than he ought to be, and contribute to the development of such increasingly common disorders as cystitis and stones (in cats), glaucoma and heart disease (in dogs), diabetes, lead poisoning, rickets, and serious vitamin-mineral deficiencies (in both cats and dogs)."

All that being said, many dog owners will still choose to feed their dogs commercial diets. Perhaps this is due to the convenience commercial foods offer, owners' doubt about challenging a veterinarian's advice and trying something new, or the very effective advertising campaigns of the pet-food industry.

The following guidelines are recommended for dog owners who choose to feed their dogs commercial diets: Avoid foods with MSG, or preserved with BHT, BTA, or ethoxyquin. Avoiding the first two may be difficult, since they are not necessarily listed on the dog food label. Seek foods that have high-quality, human-grade ingredients. Seek foods that do not have rendered fats. And, seek foods with the lowest levels of grain products.

These types of food are most often found through holistic veterinarians, holistic pet supply shops, or over the Internet. In addition, consider supplementing commercial diets with some fresh foods and digestive enzymes. (See the Suppliers section or contact your veterinarian.)

More Wholesome Options for Feeding

At this point, some readers may wish to abandon the practice of feeding commercial foods, since all kibbles share three basic problems: They are grain-based, completely processed, and laden with chemicals. Owners may have feelings of guilt or even anger regarding the information they've been given in the past. This is normal. Remember that as pet owners, we do the best we can with the information we have. The pet-food industry continues to teach consumers that dogs are only supposed to eat what comes out of a bag or a can.

Diets Prepared at Home

It is ludicrous to debate whether dogs can be maintained in good health on homemade diets. In the thousands of years since humans and dogs first began their friendship, humans have shared the food from their own hunt/farm/dining table with their dogs. It has only been in the last several decades that commercial food has been commonly available for pets. This represents an abrupt change from a diet that has lasted for centuries.

Some people are direly afraid that they will not be able to get canine nutrition "right" for their pet. The pet-food industry has convinced them that the practice of dog feeding is a complex science and that every meal must be completely and painstakingly balanced according to dubious industry standards. The concept of creating carbon-copy meals is highly artificial and even detrimental. Humans and dogs alike were designed to achieve a balanced diet *over time*. We were never designed to eat the same meals every day of our entire lives.

If commercial diets truly offered the excellent nutrition they advertise, dog owners would not be supplementing these foods with a never-ending parade of vitamins, minerals, herbs, and oils. Rather than focus on the practice of supplementing poor-quality commercial foods, this text will concentrate, instead, on the value of switching to a home-prepared diet. If you can feed yourself and your family, you can feed your dog, too.

Preparing a Home-cooked Diet

Pet owners frequently express uncertainty when switching to a home-cooked diet. They want to have hard, fast rules to follow. Feeding dogs with health problems rarely follows strict rules, however. Here are some guidelines to follow but you and your veterinarian will still need to evaluate your dog's ongoing condition, weight, and metabolism.

The most current recommendation for preparing a home-*cooked* diet is as follows:

The diet should consist of approximately 50% meat (ground meat such as beef, turkey, or chicken); organ meat, eggs, and fish, such as sardines or mackerel; as well as the occasional *cultured* milk product, such as plain yogurt or kefir.

If you chose to add grain to your dog's diet, feed no more than about one-sixth of the diet, or 15%, as grain.

The remainder, 35% to 50% should consist of vegetables and fruits, preferably pulped or blended in a food processor.

Feeding Dogs With Kidney Disease or Pancreatitis

This diet is easily adapted to dogs with special needs. If your dog suffers from pancreatitis, use lean cuts of meat. Drain away any cooked fat and grease from the meat. Remember that commercial dog food damages the GI tract early in puppyhood. This makes fat digestion difficult, if not nearly impossible, for some dogs. Add digestive enzymes to the diet. Feeding small, frequent meals may also be helpful as it places less stress on the pancreas.

Dogs suffering from kidney disease may benefit from reduced levels of protein (30% to 40%) and increased levels of the vegetable mixture (60% to 70%.) High-quality protein and the comparative lack of chemicals in homemade diets will also ease the strain on kidney function. Avoid foods high in phosphorus. (See page 94.)

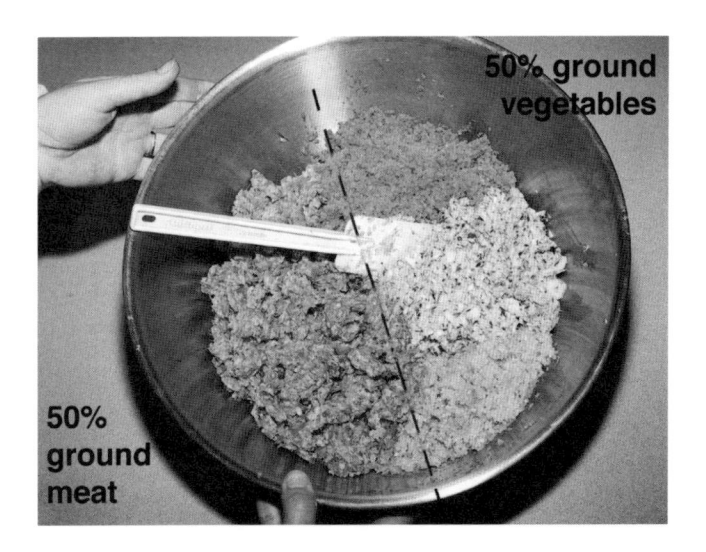

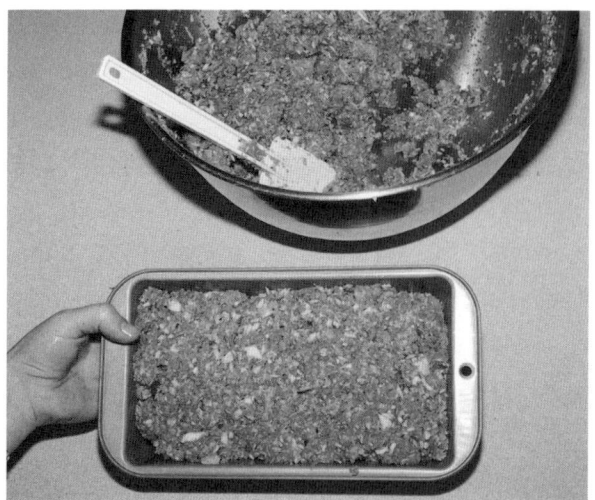

Meal preparation may seem awkward at first, but as with any habit, it becomes faster and easier with time. Most dog owners feeding home-cooked meals basically prepare a stew. Some cook the meat in a skillet, a Dutch oven/crock pot, or microwave oven. If they choose to feed grains, they cook or soak them beforehand, then add them to the cooked meat. Vegetables are finely chopped or pulped and then added to the mixture. Other owners mix together ground meat and chopped vegetables and cook them all together, resulting in the equivalent of a doggy-meatloaf.

It is possible to take an even more relaxed approach to feeding. Some owners feed a variety of foods that they themselves are eating. This may include such items as pasta with meat and tomato sauce; leftover meats such as cooked fish, roast beef, chicken (with *cooked* bones removed); leftover baked potatoes, vegetables, and overripe fruit. When leftovers are scarce, they may bake a potato and top it with a can of chicken, tuna, sardines, or a soft-boiled egg or two. (Canned tuna should be fed sparingly to epileptics, as most brands contain MSG in the form of soy or vegetable broth.)

Unless a dog exhibits a skin allergy, eggs are an excellent addition to the diet. Eggs contain omega fatty acids, which have anti-inflammatory properties and improve neural function. The protein in eggs is one of the most complete sources of essential amino acids. This includes methionine, which aids liver function and the methylation process (performing many enzymatic reactions throughout the body). Egg protein is easily digested and has a high degree of bioavailability. Eggs contain **lecithin**, a nutrient that helps emulsify dietary fat and lower cholesterol.

Many veterinarians and pet-food salesmen will frown upon this approach, and yet, it is the way in which dogs have been successfully fed for decades. Owners may notice one other important benefit of feeding this way. They may begin eating better themselves. Many people notice an improvement in their own health when they replace highly processed, heavily preserved foods with those that are whole and fresh.

Above and beyond this basic formulation (50% meat, 35% to 50% vegetables, and no more than 15% grain) there are some fine points you may wish to consider. When cooking meats, cook them lightly (rare or medium-rare). Meats cooked well-done are devoid of intrinsic enzymes. Meats can include ground meat or larger cuts, as well as organ meats such as liver, kidneys, and heart. *Always* cook salmon for dogs and remove any cooked bones. Cold-water fish, such as fatty tuna, sardines and mackerel supply fish oil and **omega fatty acids**. These are important to both neural and liver function.

If you choose to add grain to your dog's diet, consider oatmeal. Oatmeal seems to be one of the least offending grains to dogs and is an effective form of fiber in the diet. Oatmeal can be cooked, or soaked overnight in water or yogurt.

Other excellent sources of fiber include pumpkin (plain, not "pie-filling" which contains sugar). Pumpkin also helps **control diarrhea**. Celery, apples and broccoli, stems and all, are other good sources of fiber. Based on a biologically appropriate approach, large amounts of grains and bran products should be avoided. Fiber is best supplied from fruit and vegetable sources.

Dogs with excess cortisol production may exhibit a voracious appetite. The same may be true when your dog's AED dose is increased, as several have steroid-like effects. To help quench your dog's appetite, without encouraging weight gain, try low-calorie vegetables as fillers: Zucchini, celery, carrots, or green beans.

It is strongly recommended that you pulp fruits and vegetables in a blender or food processor. Dogs have difficulty breaking down the cell walls of plant material. When you break foods down mechanically, the dog's digestive system has better access to the nutrients. In addition, *do* cook such vegetables as potatoes, yams, and squash. Other vegetables can be served *either* cooked or raw.

The following vegetables are considered rather **high in sugar** and should be fed sparingly to dogs with a history of hypoglycemia, skin allergies, or obesity: Potatoes, carrots, winter squash, and green peas. The high sugar content, and resulting swings in blood sugar, may play a role in seizure activity.

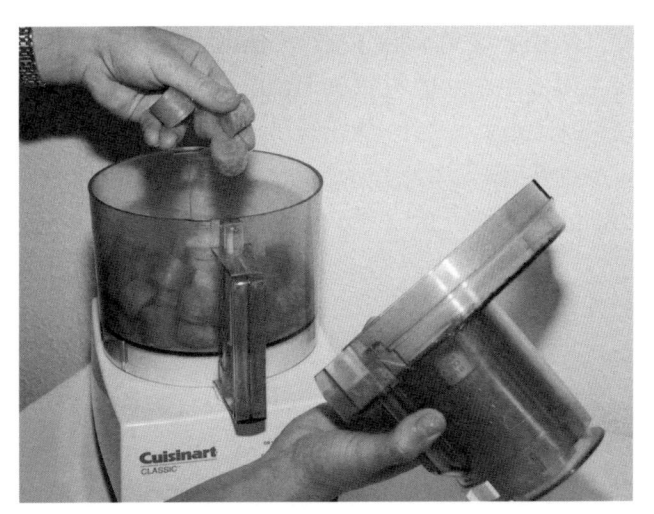

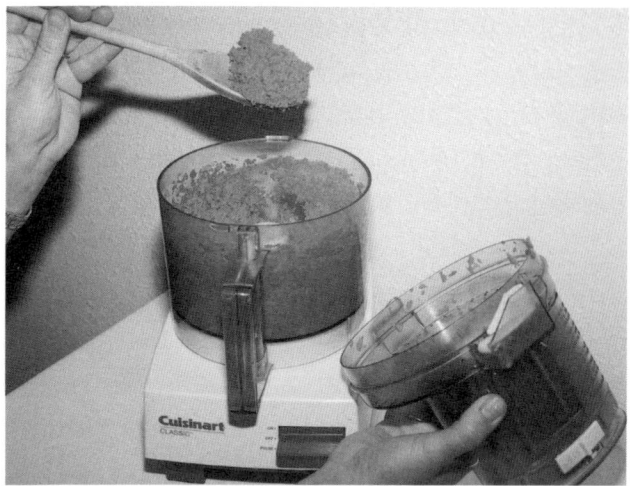

Low **sugar** vegetables include dark leafy greens such as spinach and lettuce, kale, celery, cabbage, and broccoli. These are good sources of **Vitamin E**, an antioxidant that also supports liver and neural function. Dark, leafy vegetables are also high in **magnesium**, as are apples, sunflower seeds, nuts, bananas, parsley, peanut butter, meat, and fish. Sufficient levels of magnesium may help reduce signs of weakness, irritability, insulin resistance, seizure activity and soft-tissue calcium deposits. Magnesium helps to block the entry of calcium into neurons, thereby raising the seizure threshold.

Foods such as corn, yogurt, tomatoes, beans, peas, nuts, oatmeal, sardines, bran, spinach, sweet potatoes, cheese and bananas are **high in potassium** content. Meat, yeast, grain, canned fish, nuts, eggs, and potatoes are **high in phosphorus**. Reduce the latter in cases of kidney degeneration.

Some experts recommend that certain foods should be avoided in cases of hypothyroidism. These foods produce substances known as **goitrogens**, which impair thyroid production. You may hear people cautioning against foods such as walnuts, almonds, peanuts, brussel sprouts, cauliflower, broccoli, spinach, mustard greens, and soybeans (tofu).

These recommendations stem from human healthcare circles where modern man places some unusual demands on the thyroid gland. Metabolism is stimulated in **spikes**, by stimulants such as coffee, cola, (caffeine), nicotine, and diets high in sugar. Additionally, the thyroid gland function naturally wanes as we age. Since humans live longer and longer, middle-aged humans often suffer from low or "sluggish" thyroid function. Consequently, the low-goitrogenic diet may, indeed, be helpful for some humans.

Consider again, the plight of the average dog. The most common causes of low thyroid function involve excess cortisol and/or autoimmune destruction of the thyroid gland.

Avoiding cruciferous vegetables is of little importance to autoimmune thyroid patients, since these vegetables are believed to interfere with thyroid *production*. If there are no thyroid cells, there is no production with which to interfere. However, some veterinarians still recommend this course of action since residual thyroid tissue may remain.

This illustrates the importance of having a complete picture of thyroid activity. A multiple test panel is the best way to obtain that. (See Chapter 11, *Additional Health Concerns*.) Thyroid treatment should be specific to the problem. If the autoimmune process has completely destroyed the gland (common in dogs), lifelong replacement therapy will be necessary and dietary support is less relevant. If the problem is interference by excess cortisol, reducing chronic irritants may be helpful. A less processed diet is the first step in that process.

That being said, **DO avoid soy**, tofu, and soy sauce. Whether it is classified as a protein, a bean, or a grain, soy is not biologically appropriate for the dog. Moreover, soy contains natural glutamates, the amino acid responsible for excitatory nerve transmissions.

Healthy dogs eating *cooked* diets should receive some calcium and phosphorus supplementation. If your dog suffers from alterations in calcium metabolism (see page 55), consider adding magnesium to the diet. This may help lower serum calcium levels by moving calcium back into bone and cartilage. Magnesium oxide is the most commonly available form of magnesium. However, it is difficult for the body to use. If you wish to supplement your dog's diet with magnesium, choose magnesium taurinate or magnesium citrate.

If you do add calcium and phosphorus to the diet, be advised that a certain amount of debate exists as to the best source of these minerals. Some dog owners add a 1/2 teaspoon of ground eggshells for every pound of meat. They save their eggshells, grind them in a coffee grinder, and store them in the refrigerator until needed. Some use bone meal. Others use prepared vitamin/mineral supplements available from pet supply shops and veterinarians. Also, consider supplementing fully cooked diets with **digestive enzymes**. This will help ease the workload on the pancreas.

Dog owners frequently ask, "How *much* food should I give my dog?" One rule of thumb recommends that a dog's daily food intake should equal 2% to 3% of his body-weight. Dogs are individuals, though. They have different metabolic rates. Some dogs are "high energy" individuals requiring more calories and others may have impaired thyroid function and a slower metabolic rate. The overall state of the dog's immune system will have an effect on his metabolic rate, too. In other words, dietary recommendations are simply suggestions and you may have to adjust the levels of ingredients as your dog's metabolism stabilizes.

By varying the ingredients you include, you will supply your dog with a healthy variety of nutrients. This is the way in which dogs (and people) were naturally designed to eat.

You can save yourself time and energy by making enough stew for about a week's worth of meals. Divide the stew into freezer-bag portions or small containers and freeze them. You will quickly get in the habit of taking out one bag to defrost whenever your dog finishes the previous portion.

The Benefits of Feeding Home-cooked Diets

The benefits of feeding your dog a home-cooked meal are numerous. Your dog will be ingesting few, if any, preservatives, chemicals, or dyes. He will be receiving nutrients of *much* higher quality and nutritional value, including the highly digestible amino acids and fatty acids so important for brain function. And, you can virtually eliminate grains from the diet. Homemade diets also appear to reduce the degree of cortisol symptoms.

Numerous dog owners report that homemade diets significantly reduce seizure activity and the necessary dosages of both antiseizure medications and thyroid supplements. It is unclear whether this improvement is related to lowered cortisol levels, improved cell membrane health, lower levels of chemicals, or more normal production of neurotransmitters. Whatever the case, the reports are noteworthy. Dog owners also report reduced appetite, polyuria, skin infections, diarrhea, lethargy, and muscle weakness.

The Drawbacks of Feeding Home-cooked Diets

Preparing homemade dog food may also have some drawbacks for your family. It will require more of your time. It will require more of your freezer space. And, it is likely to cost you about the same or more than premium or prescription dog foods. Offset costs by purchasing ingredients at warehouse-style grocery stores or by asking the butcher to order your dog's meat in bulk.

It is also possible for home-cooked diets to have some of the same drawbacks as commercial diets. If you cook food at high temperatures, amino acids, enzymes, fatty acids, and some vitamins will be damaged. If you choose to feed large amounts of grain, your dog may experience many of the same problems he has from eating a commercial diet.

If meals are consistently prepared in the style of a "stew" such that all the food elements (proteins, carbohydrates, fats, and minerals) are present at the same meal, some of them combine in unfortunate ways. Proteins and certain minerals can form complexes with carbohydrates and various lipids, rendering them unavailable.

And yet, even the most over-cooked, stew-style, home-prepared meal is an incredible improvement over commercial dog food. Remember, the argument still remains that for many, many years, dogs have been living long, healthy lives while sharing his owner's leftovers.

Raw Food Diets

Dog owners have another option in preparing meals at home. This is the Biologically Appropriate Raw Food diet, also known as the Bones and Raw Food diet, or BARF. This diet attempts — within limits — to reproduce the diet of the wolf and wild dog. It consists of raw meat or raw meaty bones (such as chicken necks, wings, and backs) and mostly raw fruits and vegetables.

Many pet owners are now convinced that this type of nutrition is necessary for their pets to achieve optimum health. In the 1940s, Dr. Francis Pottinger Jr. did a series of controlled studies that support this belief. His studies demonstrated that cats fed raw diets were far more healthy and resistant to disease and developmental abnormalities than cats fed the same cooked foods. Even so, the traditional veterinary community poorly accepts the BARF diet. The two most commonly cited objections are fear of feeding bones and fear of bacteria.

Remember the natural design of the dog. The teeth are designed to tear meat and crunch bones. Wild dogs routinely consume the bones of their prey as part of their meal. As Dr. Ian Billinghurst points out in his book *Give Your Dog a Bone*, it is **cooked bones**, not raw bones that cause dogs problems such as GI perforations. Cooked bones shatter and splinter. Raw bones are soft and digested by the dog's strong stomach acids.

In years past, owners commonly gave their pets raw meaty bones from their own farms, ranches, or butchers. Pet-food companies, and their strong influence in veterinary schools, have steered owners away from this practice. The omission of meaty bones from the canine diet has paralleled the development of veterinary dentistry. Dogs that chewed raw bones had **clean teeth naturally**. They did not require dental chew toys, toothbrushes, or surgical procedures with general anesthesia to maintain normal dental health.

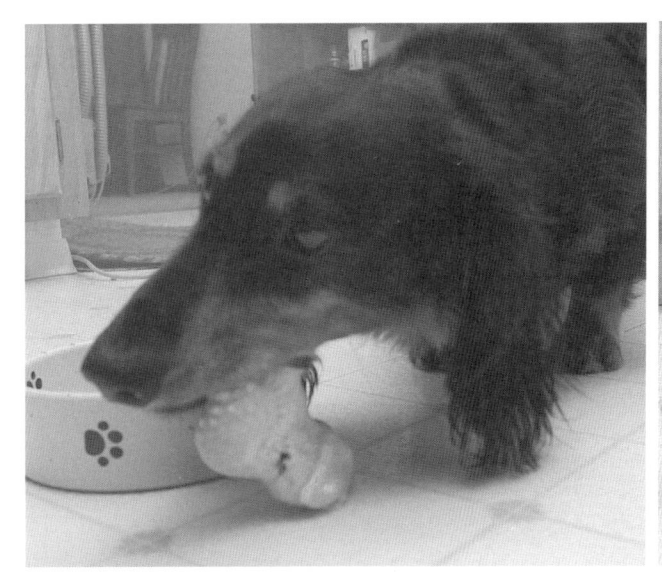

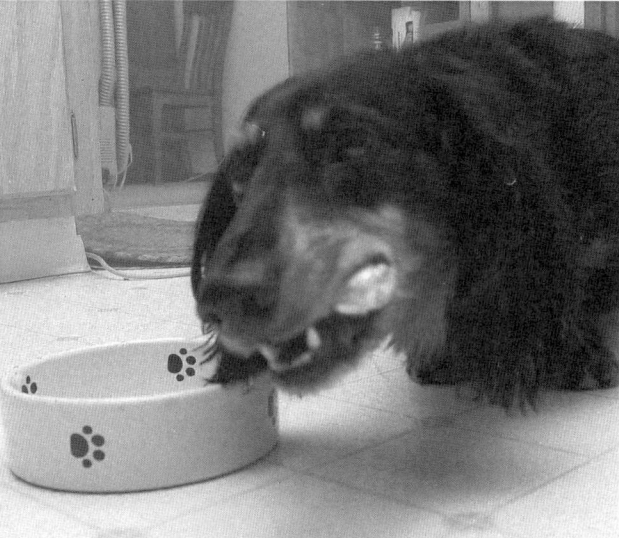

Many people have been taught to have an undue **fear of germs**. The reality is that dogs regularly come into contact with bacteria, including e-coli and salmonella, on a daily basis. Such contact is an integral part of canine behavior. It is normal for these bacteria to be present in the canine digestive tract.

Given the chance, many dogs will roll in the droppings and carcasses of other animals. Dogs will eat these things, too. They will bury chew toys in dirt, and contentedly gnaw on them later. Most common of all, dogs groom their own hind ends! Dogs come in contact with these "dangerous" bacteria all day long. Their bodies were designed to handle them. In fact, it is *important* that dogs come in contact with germs so that they develop immunity. Only dogs with weakened immune systems, or prolonged antibiotic use, face a threat from bacterial overgrowth.

Another argument you may hear opposing raw food is that "just because wolves eat a certain way, doesn't mean pet dogs should, too. After all, wild dogs die much younger than our pets do." This argument is not valid. The Grey Wolf lives an average of 10 to 12 years in the wild. Most of us know of at least one dog that died prematurely, either from cancer or other serious illness. Of the domestic dogs that *do* live longer, many are subjected to chronic, expensive, painful diseases in ever-increasing numbers.

That being said, it is important to introduce raw foods to chronically ill dogs, *slowly*. Their immune systems are already compromised. Their pancreatic function may be taxed. Their organs are inflamed. These dogs will need help in assimilating the rich supply of nutrients a fresh diet can provide.

Preparing a Raw Food Diet

There are two basic methods of preparing a BARF diet. Neither one includes much, if any, grain product. In the first method, meat meals are served separately from vegetable meals. This separation prevents various nutrients and minerals from binding together, which can render them unavailable. It also provides the kidneys with a much-needed rest. Meals consisting mainly of vegetables put little demand on kidney function.

About 50% to 70% of the diet should consist of raw meaty bones (RMBs.) These can include chicken necks, wings, or backs. RMBs are different than large joint bones. RMBs are crunched up by the dog and consumed as meals. They contain a biologically appropriate ratio of meat, calcium, and phosphorus. You may wish to remove the excess fat and skin if your dog suffers from pancreatitis or obesity.

Joint bones — also called knuckle or soup bones — also have a place in the BARF diet.

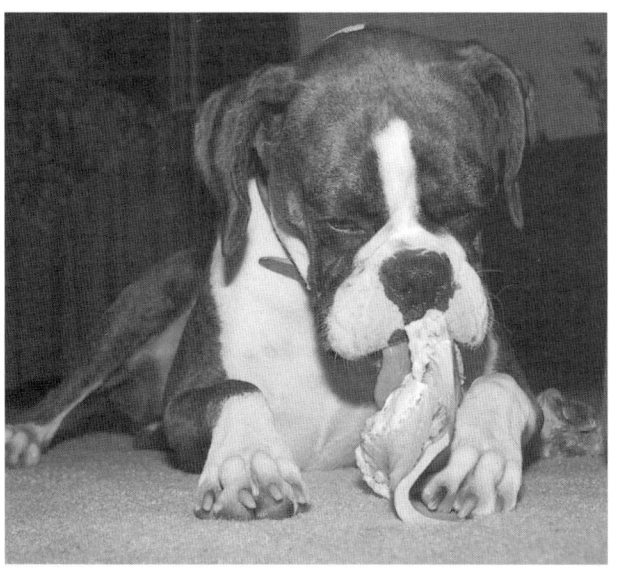

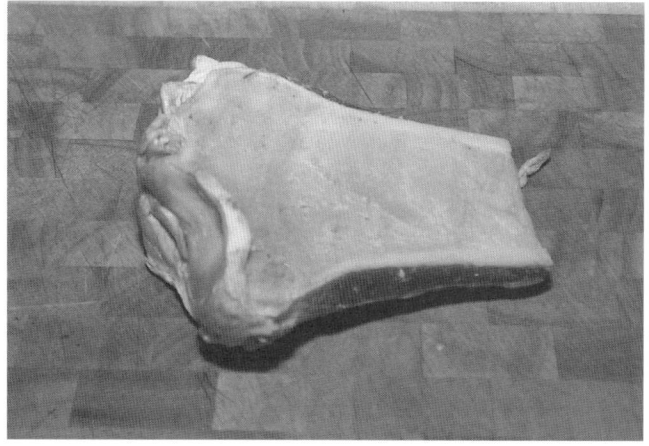

They provide an excellent way to entertain both overly energetic and lethargic dogs. Joint bones, too, should be offered raw, as cooked bones can break into dangerous shards. Throw bones away when they get small as some overly ambitious dogs might try to swallow them whole.

The second version of the raw food diet offers meat and vegetables together. In this method, RMBs may either be offered intact or passed through a meat-grinding machine. This appeals to those dog owners who simply cannot accept the idea of feeding whole bones. (See Suppliers section for commercial meat grinders.)

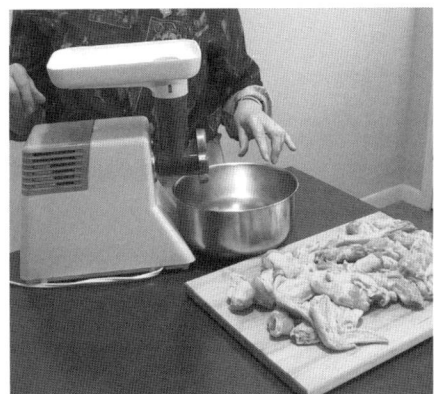

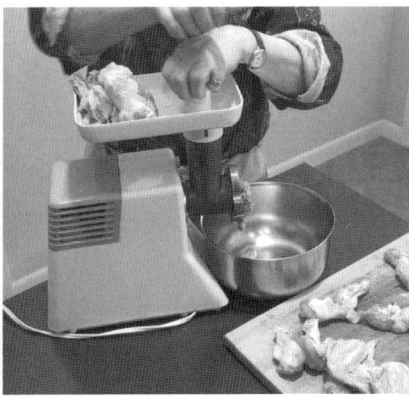

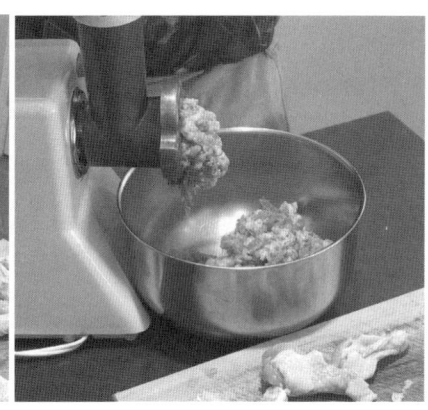

Try to include a *variety* of meats and vegetables. This provides the dog with a healthier spectrum of nutrients. This is the way humans and dogs were designed to eat—achieving balance *over time.*

Vegetable meals can actually contain a variety of things in addition to just vegetables. This includes fruit, organ meat (liver, kidney, heart), eggs, sardines, and yogurt. As previously discussed in the cooked-diet section, vegetables should be finely ground. Starchy vegetables such as potatoes, yams, and squash are actually best cooked.

If you do feed grain, cook it thoroughly or soak it overnight in warm water or yogurt. Some people feed eggs whole and raw, some soft boil them, others cook them fully. The main concern is that raw egg whites contain avidin, which in very large amounts binds with biotin, an essential B vitamin, rendering it unavailable to the body.

If you find that your dog does not enjoy his vegetable meals, try adding a small amount of garlic, tomato sauce, banana, pumpkin, or ground meat (especially liver) in the mixture. Some dog owners add as much as 50% ground meat (muscle meat or organ meat) to the vegetable mixture. Most dogs find these ingredients highly palatable.

Do *not* add calcium supplements to BARF diets. The raw meaty bones will supply appropriate levels of calcium and other minerals. Added supplements may actually cause joint and skeletal problems.

As with cooked diets, it is possible to prepare meals as your schedule permits and freeze the excess. You will quickly get into the habit of defrosting one container each time you feed your dog. Freezing fresh food does not damage intrinsic enzymes but may damage the water-soluble vitamins (C and B vitamins) to some degree.

Running warm water over RMBs will help bring them to room temperature before serving. When veggie meals are frozen in plastic containers or plastic bags, they can be thawed in a bowl of hot water.

The Benefits of Feeding Raw Food Diets

Feeding your dog fresh, raw foods will supply him with undamaged and intact amino acids, vitamins, minerals, and enzymes. Raw calories are less stimulating to the pituitary gland and the appetite center in the brain. This helps reduce symptoms of hunger. It helps stabilize body weight. Of all the dietary options, fresh, raw diets, without grains, require the least amount of insulin.

Preparing raw food meals typically takes less time than making home-cooked meals (since no cooking is required). They are also more economical since the meaty bones (chicken necks, wings, and backs) are less costly than ground meat or filets.

Fresh foods contain intact enzymes, greatly reducing stress on the exocrine pancreas. Dogs process this food quickly. Less energy is engaged in digestion and can be diverted to other activities, such as immune system function. Biologically appropriate foods are less irritating to the intestinal tract. They place much less stress on kidney and liver function, as well. Like home-cooked diets, fresh food can reduce the required levels of AEDs and thyroid supplements.

The Drawbacks of Feeding Raw Food Diets

As with the any diet, the BARF diet does have its drawbacks. It is more time consuming than feeding commercial diets. (See Suppliers section for commercially prepared BARF diets.) It requires as much, or more, freezer space as home-cooked diets. If you board your dog at a kennel, or hire a dog-sitter, others may be uncomfortable or unwilling to feed raw food. In these cases, it may be best to provide containers of cooked food for the time you'll be away. And finally, your veterinarian may not be supportive of this concept.

Variations in Homemade Diets

Several variations are possible in the preparation of homemade diets. Some dog owners choose to cook all the ingredients in the diet. Some cook the meat and the grain, leaving the vegetables fresh; others choose to cook the meat only, very lightly. Variations also exist in raw food diets. Some owners do not feed bones, until cortisol (and calcium) levels are brought under control. (See page 55.) Dogs without calcium problems and eating no bones may be fed calcium supplements.

NOTE: Some human epileptic children are treated using a **ketogenic diet**. This is a diet low in carbohydrates and high in dietary fat. In humans, this diet results in the body's production of ketones, which may help some patients, particularly children, avoid seizures. However, dogs do not metabolize ketones in the same manner, therefore, the ketogenic diet is not recommended for use in dogs. Preparing a biologically appropriate diet may indeed be the best approach to epilepsy and a host of other health problems.

Switching Diets

Whether you are switching your dog from one commercial diet to another, or from commercial to homemade, two things apply. It should be done gradually and it should be done with your veterinarian's knowledge. Make the switch over many weeks. Some individuals may take months. These dogs are likely to have irritated organs throughout their bodies.

Homemade meals (cooked or fresh) can result in the need for *much lower* levels of AED's, especially potassium bromide. This stems from the fact that commercial food contains table salt (sodium chloride). Both potassium bromide and sodium chloride are salts and interact with the body in similar ways. In fact, they *compete* with each other.

Bromide and chloride compete for the chance to be excreted by the kidneys. Perhaps more importantly, they also compete for uptake by the GI tract. When high levels of sodium chloride are present, there is less "space" from which potassium bromide can be absorbed. Diets high in sodium (commercial food) result in lower circulating levels of KBr. Conversely, the switch to a low salt diet (homecooked and BARF diets) may result in KBr levels that are suddenly too high for your dog.

Switching from commercial food to homemade food can reduce the necessary KBr dosage by as much as 50% in some dogs. The reduction can be seen quickly, sometimes, in just a matter of days. You may wish to have levels of both KBr *and Pb* checked as you make the switch. Be alert for signs of overmedication, such as ataxia (loss of muscle coordination), lethargy, increased thirst, and urination. If you observe these signs, contact your veterinarian and discuss reducing your dog's dose. Appetite may increase simply because the food is more palatable and may not be as reliable an indicator of excess medication levels.

Since sodium chloride is not necessarily listed on commercial food labels, a telephone call to the manufacturing company may be in order. Contact the makers of both the pet food you're removing from the dog's diets, as well as the makers of the new pet food. Ask them to supply you with information regarding the levels of chloride (sodium chloride) in their products.

The change in diet can also affect the way the dog's body uses nutrients and stores fat. Monitor weight gain and weight loss. Adjust meal size accordingly. Because "real" food is more nutrient-rich, a dog may require a smaller total portion than the commercial food he was eating. Keep your veterinarian apprised of your plans and progress.

To switch from one commercial diet to another commercial diet, exchange a few of the regular kibble for the new kibble, or a spoonful of the regular canned food for the new canned food. Each day, add a bit more of the new food and less of the old food. This process should be accomplished slowly, over the course of several weeks. If the new food has higher levels of sodium chloride, your dog may require an increase in his KBr dose. If the new food has lower levels, your dog may require a reduction in KBr.

To switch from a commercial diet to any type of homemade diet, progress especially slowly. Remember that your dog may have compromised immune, endocrine, and metabolic function in addition to his seizure problems.

Dogs living on commercial diets for long periods may have inflamed internal organs and absorption problems. They may require extra help in digesting new foods. So even if you are adding fresh (raw) food that contains intrinsic enzymes, strongly consider adding digestive enzymes to this diet while your dog first adjusts. These are available at pet supply shops (see Suppliers list) or through veterinarians. Dietary enzymes may help in the metabolism of fat-soluble vitamins and essential fatty acids so necessary for neural health.

Begin the switch by adding meat first (whichever you decide, raw or cooked). Add small amounts until a ratio of 50% meat to 50% commercial food is reached. Then add the vegetable/mix, a spoonful at a time. Following that step, add any grain products, *if* you choose to do so. As you increase the volume of homemade food, decrease the volume of commercial food.

Since both homecooked and BARF diets will be significantly lower in sodium chloride, KBr doses will likely need to be readjusted. Dog owners report a reduction of as much as 50% in necessary KBr levels. This may also be due to less irritating nature of homemade food, resulting in lower levels of circulating cortisol.

To switch a dog to the BARF diet, introduce raw meaty bones (chicken necks, wings, or backs) separately from kibble meals. Kibble and raw meaty bones digest quite differently and it is recommended that they not be fed at the same time. Gradually replace 50% to 70% of the kibble meals with RMB meals. Then introduce ground veggie/organ meat/egg, etc. meals to make up the remainder.

Snacks, Treats, and How to Hide Medications

If you are feeding a commercial diet, seek out treats that have the lowest levels of grain and highest levels of meat. Avoid treats containing high levels of corn (some synthetic chew bones), wheat, rice (rice cakes), and soy (tofu). As previously discussed, dogs are not designed to assimilate these ingredients. Avoid commercial biscuits and treats that have high levels of sugar.

If you are feeding a homemade diet, you can use a variety of real foods as snacks. Many dogs are fond of raw carrots, bananas, or apples. Raw foods do not raise blood sugar levels as much as cooked foods do. (There is a tendency to believe that adding sugary foods to the diet will help supply glucose to brain cells. This may prove unhelpful if insulin production is already exhausted from a diet high in carbohydrates and sugars. In these cases, adding sugar to the diet is useless to brain cells.)

Other owners offer small amounts of protein, such as a slice of turkey meat or roast beef. (Avoid the chemically laden, prepackaged type.) Some owners even prepare homemade meat jerky. This can be made from beef or boneless chicken breasts sliced thinly. Garlic powder can be added for extra flavor. The meat is placed in a dehydrator or oven set at 145 degrees F overnight or for most of the day. Avoid marinating the meat in soy sauce or other sauces containing soy, as they are a source of the excitatory NT glutamate. Also

Chapter 8 — Dietary Therapy 105

avoid salting the meat, as it can interfere with KBr absorption. Instead, refrigerate unused portions after dehydrating.

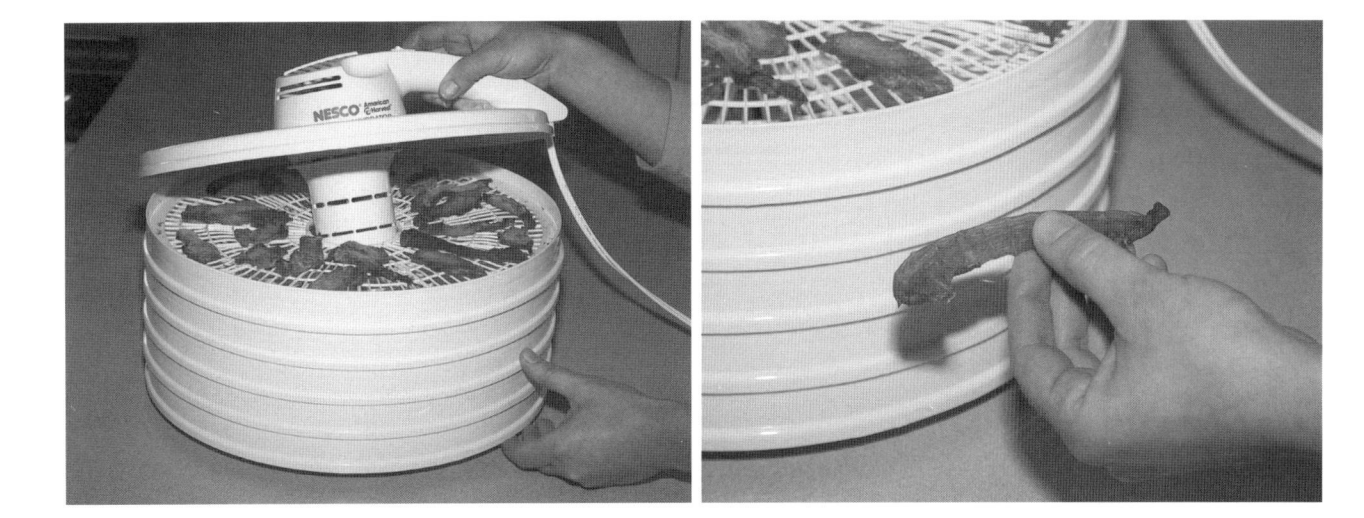

Oral medications or supplements can be hidden inside folded pieces of luncheon meat. If your dog has transitioned to a raw food diet, you may find chicken hearts to be an excellent vehicle for dispensing pills. (They have a perfect pill-sized cavity.) For very finicky eaters, try hiding pills in cream cheese, liverwurst, or tuna fish. While some of these are higher in fat content, they may help get medication down in worst-case scenarios.

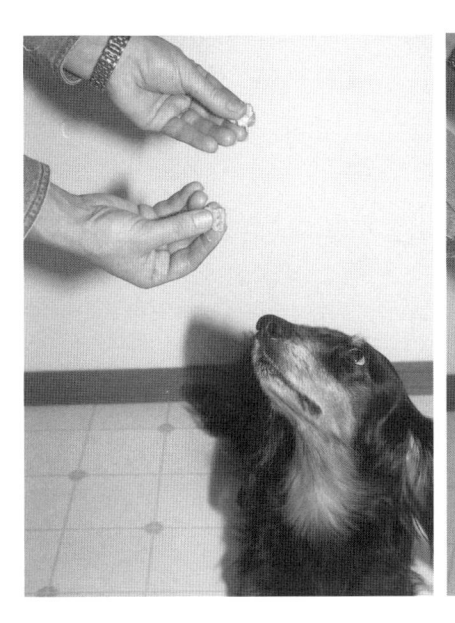

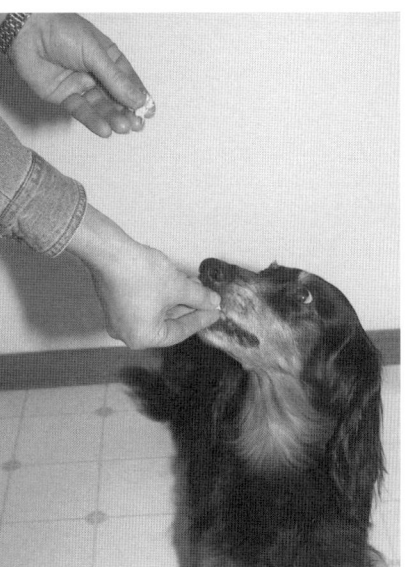

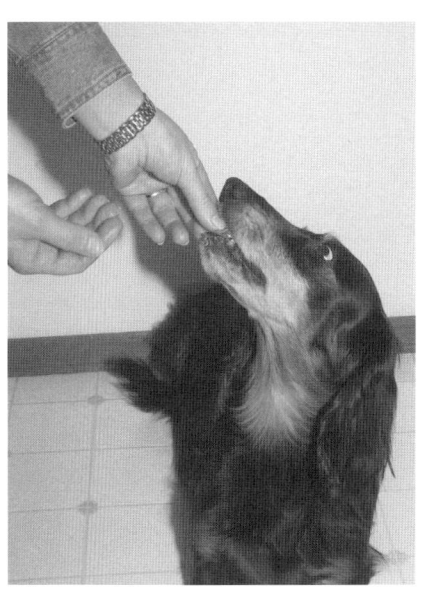

Regardless of the food treat, the **rapid-fire method** is very successful way to medicate dogs. This involves feeding a food treat (with the pill hidden inside) and *immediately* offering a second food treat (without a pill). Dogs are usually so interested in getting the second treat that they readily swallow the first one without taking time to sort out the medication. Build the trust of finicky eaters by offering them a plain treat *prior* to the medicated treat.

Dogs with excess cortisol production may exhibit a voracious appetite. The same may be true when your dog's level of AEDs is increased, as several have steroid-like effects. This may persist for several weeks. For voracious eaters, try offering low-calorie, high-fiber snacks such as carrots, celery, or raw beef knuckle bones. They will help distract your dog and fill his stomach for a while. Offer small, frequent meals or snacks to dogs that experience hypoglycemia. A bedtime snack may be helpful if your dog has a history of seizing during the night.

Since many snack foods made for *human* consumption are heavily laden with chemicals, it is best to avoid these, too, for your epileptic dog. Such items would include snack chips, prepackaged luncheon meats, hot dogs, and beef jerky. As you begin to read labels, you will see just how many chemicals are used in the food industry.

Water Consumption

It is always important to provide dogs with ample water, but especially so if a dog is experiencing symptoms of excess cortisol production or steroid effects. Some dog owners are tempted to restrict a dog's water consumption to reduce urinary accidents but this can have dire consequences. Limiting water intake does *not* reduce urination. Instead, it may result in dehydration. This is a serious situation that can lead to increased seizure activity and even death. These dogs need access to unlimited water. Frequently check the water bowl.

Changes in Body Weight

Changes in body weight are common as various metabolic problems are brought under control. Supplying dogs with more wholesome and biologically appropriate nutrition may result in improved metabolism and some weight gain. Dogs switched to homemade meals may not need the same volume of food as when they were fed commercial food.

If your dog is obese, weight loss should be achieved slowly over a period of several months. Reducing fats and grains in the diet and introducing fresh foods should contribute to weight loss. Less irritation and lower cortisol levels may also increase your dog's interest in physical activity.

Dietary Supplements

Dog owners add countless dietary supplements to commercial pet food in an attempt to improve it. To examine the full extent of these products is beyond the scope of this book. This author believes that it is healthier to improve the basic diet. In addition, the body (both human and canine) was designed to utilize nutrients in their natural forms, combinations, and potencies. Some concern exists as to whether supplying individual nutrients does more harm than good.

All that being said, there *are* a few oral supplements that may be worthy of your consideration. Since commercial food is suspected to damage the intestinal tract of puppies, dogs raised on commercial food may have difficulty absorbing nutrients even after a switch to the most natural and wholesome diet. In addition, cortisol and antiepileptic drugs are known to lower tissue levels of Vitamin C, Vitamin E, and the B vitamins.

Vitamins, Minerals, and Antioxidants

The B vitamins — are necessary for GABA production and can be depleted in humans taking AEDs. The most efficient method of supplying B vitamins is in the form of Vitamin B "complex." This provides the range of B vitamins in appropriate proportions.

In his article "Seizure Disorder in Cats and Dogs," Dr. Roger Clemmons recommends supplementing with one "regular" formula B vitamin complex pill or gelcap daily for small dogs, one "high-potency B 50" for medium dogs, and one "stress formula B 100" for large dogs.

Vitamin E — has antiseizure and anti-inflammatory properties. It reduces free radical damage to cell membranes. (It also reduces platelet stickiness.) Vitamin E levels are often reduced by antiepileptic medications. Dr. Clemmons recommends vitamin E at a rate of 400 to 800 IU per day. Vitamin C and selenium work in concert with Vitamin E.

Vitamin C — Dr. Clemmons recommends Vitamin C at 250 to 500 mg, bid (twice daily).

Trace minerals — **Selenium** works synergistically with Vitamin E. It is necessary to create the enzyme glutathione peroxidase, which protects nerve cell membranes from the damage of free radical molecules. It is found in broccoli, cabbage, fish, and meat. These, along with apples, spinach, and peanut butter, are good sources of **zinc** and **manganese**, two other trace minerals that are important for neural health.

Calcium and phosphorus — supplementation levels depend on the type of meals your dog is receiving. Dogs eating raw bone diets should not be fed any calcium supplements. Some owners of dogs eating cooked diets, or raw diets *without* bones, add 1/2 teaspoon of ground eggshells for every pound of meat. They save their eggshells, grind them in a coffee grinder and store them in the refrigerator until needed. Some use bone meal. Others use prepared vitamin/mineral supplements available from pet supply shops and veterinarians.

Magnesium — plays a large role in raising the seizure threshold. It helps close calcium channels in the neurons, thereby protecting the cell from excess firing and membrane damage. Magnesium helps to recycle homocysteine in the methylation process and it helps deposit calcium into bone, ligament, and cartilage where it belongs. In addition, some researchers believe that zinc and magnesium suppress a phenomenon known as neuronal burst firing.

Magnesium oxide is the most commonly available magnesium supplement, however, the body poorly absorbs it. Purchase instead, magnesium citrate, magnesium ascorbate or magnesium taurinate. Some canine nutritionists warn against mineral supplement, as the addition of one mineral may adversely affect levels of other minerals. If you are of the same opinion, add magnesium-rich foods to the diet, instead. Foods high in magnesium include dark, leafy vegetables, apples, sunflower seeds, nuts, bananas, parsley, peanut butter, meat, and fish.

N-Acetylcystein — another antioxidant believed to stimulate glutathione peroxidase function and protect nerve cell membranes from the damage of free radical molecules. It has been known to cause stomach upset in some individuals.

Amino Acids

Tuarine — is considered to be a long-lasting anticonvulsant, but which is excreted through the urine in times of stress. It acts by stabilizing nerve cell membranes. Dr. Roger Kendall (in *Complimentary and Alternative Veterinary Medicine*) recommends dosing dogs with 200 to 1,000 mg per day. Magnesium taurinate supplies both taurine and magnesium.

Dimethylglycine (DMG)—is involved with metabolism at the cellular level. DMG helps in the delivery, absorption, and assimilation of oxygen, and consequently ATP production, inside each cell. Dr. Kendall recommends between 50 to 500 mg per day.

Essential Fatty Acids (EFAs)

Omega 6 fatty acids — are abundant in raw food diets and, therefore, may not require supplementing. The exception some sources recommend for epileptics is **Gamma-Linoleic Acid (GLA)**. This can be found in borage, primrose, and black current oil. Dr. Clemmons recommends GLA at a dose of 500 mg, once daily for small to medium dogs and 500 mg/bid (*twice* daily) for large dogs.

Omega 3 fatty acids — including **Docosahexaenoic Acid (DHA)**, are less abundant in the diet. Omega 3 fatty acids are available in red meat, organ meat, eggs, dark green vegetables, mackerel, and sardines. They are available in supplements such as flaxseed oil and salmon oil, which may be given several times weekly. Cold pressed, flaxseed oil is available in the refrigerator section of health food stores. Dr. Lew Olson recommends adding 1 teaspoon daily for small dogs and 1 tablespoon for large dogs. Occasionally, dogs may exhibit an allergic reaction to flax seed oil. Discontinue use in this case. Salmon or fish oil may be added several times weekly at a rate of 1,000 mg per 20 *pounds* of bodyweight.

S-adenosylmethionine (SAMe)

SAMe is a compound the body produces from methionine, one of the sulfer-based essential amino acids, and ATP. SAMe produces methyl groups that are responsible for a host of normal metabolic process including the regulation of numerous hormones, neurotransmitters, cellular membranes and waste products, and even genetic predispositions. Levels of SAMe are lowered by poor metabolic function, stress, and aging.

Denosyl SD4 is a form of SAMe available through veterinarians. The manufacturer of this product recommends that dogs be dosed at the following rates:

> Dogs less than 12 pounds: one 90 mg tablet
> Dogs between 12 and 25 pounds: two 90 mg tablets
> Dogs between 25 and 35 pounds: one 225 mg tablet
> Dogs between 35 and 65 pounds: two 225 mg tablets
> Dogs over 65 pounds: three 225 mg tablets

Milk Thistle (Silymarin)

A number of studies indicate that this herb stimulates protein synthesis and regeneration of the liver. It is considered safe for use in both dogs and humans and is frequently recommended for dogs taking AEDs. It is available at health food stores and through the Internet. Milk thistle is dispensed in drops or powder dispensed in milligrams. Dr. Russell Swift recommends dosing dogs according to their weight. (Consider the dosing instructions on the label to be appropriate for a 100 to 150 pound human.)

Medicinal herbs may work best when they are given at intermittent intervals. Your veterinarian may recommend that you give the herb for five days, and then skip two days. This pattern may continue for a month or two, followed by a week's rest without any milk thistle. Then the cycle may be repeated.

Glandular Extracts

Holistic veterinarians sometimes recommend the addition of glandular extracts or "glandulars" (concentrates of raw animal glands) to the diet. The theory behind glandular extracts is that "cells help like cells." Pancreas, thymus, adrenal, and thyroid glandulars are commercially available to the veterinary community, and in some nutritional supplements. (See Suppliers list.)

Little scientific data exists on the validity of glandular extracts, but it is interesting to note that studies done at the beginning of the 20th century indicated that human diabetic patients benefited from the oral ingestion of animal pancreas extracts. Eventually, this work led scientists to the discovery and widespread use of injectable insulin, today's most common treatment of Type 1 diabetes.

Melatonin

Veterinary interest is mounting in melatonin, a hormone normally produced in the pineal gland, but also available as an oral supplement. Melatonin has been used to treat a variety of problems, including insomnia, bilateral flank alopecia (hair loss), thyroid disease, obesity, cancer, and immune deficiency disorders. Veterinarians have also recommended melatonin for neurological and behavioral issues such as aggression, separation anxiety, fear of loud noises, and epilepsy, as it is believed to increase GABA levels in the brain.

Phosphatidyl Serine (or Phosphatidylserine)

Some holistic veterinarians also prescribe the oral supplement Phosphatidyl Serine (PS) in cases of excess cortisol production and epilepsy. PS is a natural phospholipid that is normally made by the body through a series of complex processes. Levels deteriorate, however, with age and stress. PS improves nervous system and memory function in humans and raises circulating levels of hormones such as dopamine and melatonin. This, in turn, *reduces* levels of ACTH and cortisol.

Since neuronal membranes are comprised mainly of phospholipids, Phosphatidyl Serine is also important to normal brain activity. Phosphatidyl Serine keeps cell membranes supple and permeable. This may help oxygen and nutrients move more easily into brain cells. It may also help maintain normal neurotransmitter activity.

Phosphatidyl Serine was originally tested on dogs prior to FDA approval for use in humans. Adverse effects were not noted in these dogs after prolonged use on high doses. The average dose for *human* use is 300 mg per day. The owners of small dogs (weighing 10 to 25 pounds) have reported reduced symptoms of cortisol with 50 mg to 100 mg per day. The owner's of medium-size dogs (weighing 40 to 50 pounds) have reported good results with 200 mg per day. Reduced symptoms are often noted in two to three weeks. Consider administering PS in the morning — before noon — if your dog has symptoms of restlessness or insomnia in the evening. This approach will give the PS the maximum time to help reduce cortisol levels by evening.

While PS is available at most health food stores and does not require a doctor's prescription, it is still wise to keep your veterinarian apprised of your plans. If a dog is at a point where he is passing from the alarm phase (the period of excess cortisol production) to the phase of adrenal exhaustion (the period of insufficient cortisol production), the use of Phosphatidyl Serine *may* unmask that transition. If your dog demonstrates a loss of appetite or increased lethargy, discontinue the use of PS.

Digestive Enzymes

Since commercial dog food can exhaust pancreatic enzyme production and damage the intestine's ability to absorb nutrients, supplementing with digestive enzymes can be quite helpful. Digestive enzymes are made from either pancreatin, a synthetic product extracted from bovine sources, or plant sources. Since liver function — including bile production — is often compromised in epileptic dogs, it can be helpful to add digestive enzymes that included ox bile. Bile is important in digesting dietary fat. Prescription brands, and those prepared from animal sources, are typically more concentrated than are those available over the counter. Certain holistic supply houses now offer stronger preparations available to the public. (See Suppliers section.)

Most of these preparations are offered in a powdered form that is sprinkled on the dog's food. Tablets are also available. These may be more cost-effective but they may be more labor-intensive, since tablets must be crushed to work well.

Summary

It may take several weeks, a month, or more for dietary changes and supplements to take effect. It is impossible to instruct the reader as to which supplements might help his individual dog. An understanding of the disease process, supplied by this text, and a discussion with a trusted veterinarian are good starting points.

Canine nutrition is an area of considerable controversy and the veterinary community admits that not all dietary issues are well understood. For a diet to be successful, however, it must make both the animal and owner happy. If you have strong feelings about trying a new diet, it is helpful to find a veterinarian who will support you in this pursuit. You can ask the staff of a prospective veterinary clinic how the doctor feels about home-prepared or raw food diets.

Even though damage to the digestive tract occurs early in a dog's life, the body can patch a failing metabolic system. It can take years for the extent of the damage to become apparent. With the advent of each additional health problem, dog owners may mistakenly conclude that the new, more wholesome diet is responsible. Likewise, they may not believe the new diet is helpful if it doesn't improve matters immediately. While some dogs experience improved neurological function in a matter of days, it can take six months or more to ease the damage caused by a lifetime of eating commercial food.

Will a homemade diet *cure* epilepsy? Perhaps, not. Many veterinarians go by the old adage, "once a seizure dog, always a seizure dog" and intestinal damage done early in life may still result in health problems. However, a more wholesome, appropriate diet *is* likely to aid immune system function, reduce inflammation and its clinical signs, improve quality of life, and add to a dog's longevity. In numerous cases, homemade food appears to have significantly reduced or eliminated seizures and AEDs.

Allow at least a month's time before deciding whether a new diet is working for a your dog. Pets suffering from pancreatitis and inflammatory bowel syndrome may require *many* months to make the transition. Make this time as easy as possible for your dog, using a gradual approach, high-quality ingredients, and digestive enzyme supplements.

This brings up a final important point. Since it is difficult to know *which* dietary supplements might be helpful to a particular dog, and since the whole topic can be confusing and time consuming for owners, it is important to remember the basic theory of canine nutrition. Dogs that are fed a variety of unprocessed foods over time, will obtain balance and necessary nutrients.

References

Animal Protection Institute of America, Sacramento, California, "Pet Food Investigative Report," www.api4animals.org/petfood.htm, May, 1996.

Billinghurst, I., *Give Your Dog a Bone: The Practical Commonsense Way to Feed Dogs For a Long Healthy Life*, self-published: Australia, 1993.

Blaylock, R.L., *Excitotoxins: The Taste That Kills*. Santa Fe: Health Press, 1994.

Clemmons, R.M., "Seizure Disorders in Dogs and Cats," http://pawcare.com/rclemmons, January, 2002.

Dakshinamurti, K., et al, "Neuroendocrinology of Pyridoxine Deficiency," *Neuroscience and Biobehavioral Reviews*, 12: 1988.

Garcia, M.C., et al, "Effect of Docosahesaenoic Acid on the Synthesis of Phosphatidylserine in Rat Brain Microsomes and c6 Glioma Cells," *Journal of Neurochemistry*, 70(1): January, 1998.

Giroud, M., and Dumas, R., "Epilepsy and Endocrine Modifications," Encephale, March-April, 1988.

Goldstein, M., *The Nature of Animal Healing: The Path to Your Pet's Health, Happiness and Longevity*: New York: Alfred A. Knopf, 1999.

Kendall, R.V., *Complementary and Alternative Veterinary Medicine: Principles and Practice*. St. Louis: Mosby, 1997.

Levin, C.D., *Dogs, Diet and Disease: An Owner's Guide to Diabetes Mellitus, Pancreatitis, Cushing's Disease, and More.* Oregon City: Lantern Publications, 2001.

Lindenbaum, E.S., and Mueller, J.J., "Effects of Pyridoxine on Mice After Immobilization Stress," *Nutrition and Metabolism*, 17: 1974.

Martin, A.N., *Foods Pets Die For: Shocking Facts About Pet Food.* Troutdale, OR: New Sage Press, 1997.

Olson, L., "Introduction to Essential Fatty Acids and Their Use in Diet," *B-Naturals Newsletter*, December, 2001.

Osiecki, H., *The Physician's Handbook of Clinical Nutrition.* Kelvin Grove, Australia: Bio Concepts Publishing, 1995.

Plechner, A.J., and Zucker, M., *Pet Allergies: Remedies for an Epidemic.* Inglewood, CA: Very Healthy Enterprises, 1986.

Richard, A., and Reiter, J., *Epilepsy: A New Approach.* New York: Prentice Hall, 1990.

Sarjeant, D., and Evans, K., *Hard to Swallow: The Truth About Food Additives.* Burnaby, Canada: Alive Books, 1999.

Schoen, A.M., "Seizures in Dogs & Cats: An Integrative Approach with Natural Options," www.drschoen.com/articles_L2_14_.html, December, 2001.

Schultz, K.R., *The Ultimate Diet: Natural Nutrition for Dogs and Cats.* Decanso, California: Affenbar Ink, 1998.

Shames, R., and Shames K.H., *Thyroid Power: Ten Steps to Total Health.* New York: Harper Resource, 2001.

Sudha, K., et al, "Oxidative Stress and Antioxidants in Epilepsy," *Clinica Chimica Acta* 303(1-2): January, 2001.

Swift, R., "Milk Thistle: Herbal Wonder," *The Pet Tribune*, an online newsletter, http://www.pettribune.com/1998/040598/9.html, April, 1998.

Wellington, K., and Jarvis, B., "Silymarin: A Review of its Clinical Properties in the Management of Hepatic Disorders," *BioDrugs*, 15(7): 2001.

Chapter 9

Alternative Therapies

Acupuncture

Acupuncture is a 5,000-year-old tradition rooted in the philosophies of Eastern (Chinese) medicine. It revolves around the concepts of energy and the flow of that energy through the body. In the case of epilepsy, energy is believed to well up like a great wind.

The application of pressure to — or stimulation of — certain points on the body has proven helpful for some epileptics. Veterinarians trained in acupuncture can perform treatments in the clinic. These sessions are performed while your dog is awake. Various points are typically stimulated with tiny acupuncture needles or laser light in order to return energy flow to a more normal and natural pattern.

Some dogs require more permanent or constant forms of stimulation. This can be achieved when the practitioner implants tiny gold beads (1/16th inch diameter) or gold wire at the necessary pressure points. This procedure is performed under general anesthesia. According to Terry Durkes DVM, a leader in this field, improvement may be seen within a week. He reports that over half the dogs receiving this treatment will experience a reduction in seizures or required levels of Phenobarbital.

Some owners have realized the benefits of acu*pressure* performed at home. This involves gently rubbing an area on the top of the dog's head (the GV20 point) known for its calming effects. The location of this point is often marked by a slight depression in the skull. Dog owners may gently stimulate this area in an effort to elicit a more natural and normal flow of energy.

Doctors at the University of Florida College of Veterinary Medicine have identified two additional acupuncture points that have relevance to canine epilepsy. Stimulation of two points located on the ears, named Shen Men 1 and Shen Men 2, have been reported effective in reducing the extent and frequency of seizures. While the results of treatment are reported only by testimonial, veterinarians recommend it for use on all epilepsy cases since it is without harmful side effects.

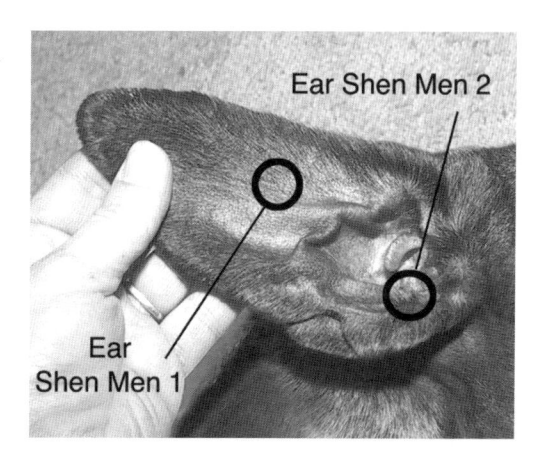

Massage

Massage may also be a useful tool in minimizing seizure activity. Human epilepsy patients demonstrate greater muscle tension than non-epileptics. This may be one marker of increased stress and higher than average cortisol levels. Some dog owners perform therapeutic massage as a way to help their dogs *recover* from a seizure, as well.

Massage can be performed daily, if you have the time. But even massage done just twice weekly is effective in lowering cortisol levels in humans. If your dog tends to seize at night, massage before bedtime might help him.

Since massage therapy deals with energy, make certain that you are in a peaceful state of mind before you begin. Try to free your mind from stressful thoughts. Breath slowly, deeply, and evenly. Massage can be a mutually enjoyable activity and a pleasant way to bond with your dog.

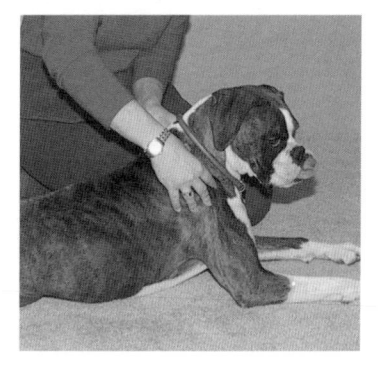

Start by stroking from the bridge of his nose and over the top of his head. Work down his neck, back, and toward his tail. As you massage pay attention to your dog's reaction. He may provide feedback as to areas that he most enjoys having massaged. If he slinks down, avoids the motion, or rolls over as if to hide an area of his body, it may be a sign of discomfort. Avoid such areas. Finish off the massage by gently rubbing his ears.

Tellington-Touch

Tellington-Touch (abbreviated TTouch) is another hands-on treatment modality that has benefits for epileptic dogs. The theory behind this method is quite unique, however. The Tellington-Touch system (developed by Linda Tellington-Jones) is based upon the concept that cells hold emotions. Certainly, prior discussions in this text illustrate that hormones and neurochemicals have distinct physiological effects at the cellular level.

Chapter 9 — Alternative Therapies   117

Unlike massage however, TTouch does not target specific areas of the body. It is not involved with loosening tight muscles. Instead, TTouch stimulates the body in "non-habitual" ways.

Dogs and humans each receive certain nerve transmissions so frequently, that they become ingrained or habitual. A good example of this is how we no longer notice the presence (the stimulation) of a favorite wristwatch. If you put on a new piece of jewelry, however, it is very noticeable. Habitual stimulations include the activities of daily life.

TTouch operates under the concept that it is possible to release the damaging effects — of emotions or stress — by stimulating the body in a non-habitual ways. One method involves stimulating random areas on the dog's body with a circular motion of the fingers. The randomness, as well as the circular motion of the skin, is unlike any habitual stimulation the dog receives in daily life.

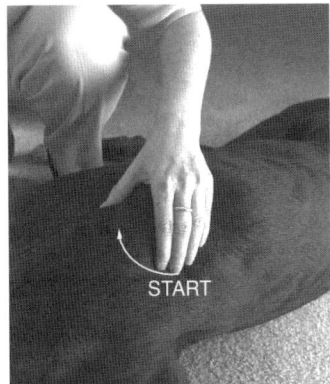

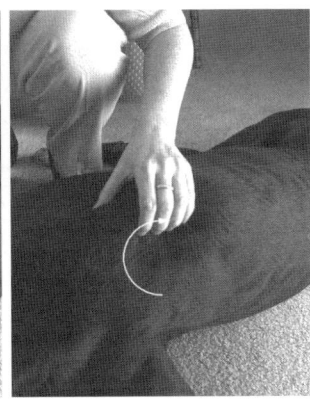

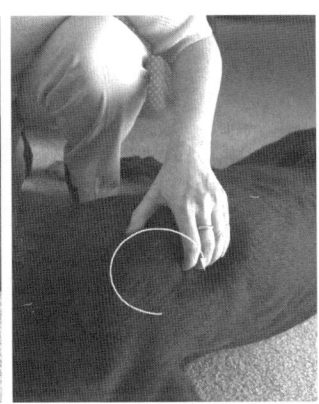

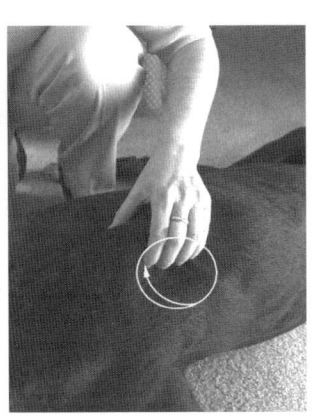

To perform TTouch, hold your hand (palm down) in a slightly cupped position. Stabilize your hand by gently resting your thumb on the dog's body. Using light pressure move your fingers in a one-and-one-quarter, circular motion. Circle clockwise. Then lift your hand and move it to another random area of the body.

TTouch pressure should be firm enough to rotate the skin but it should not lift and massage deep, muscle tissue. Remember, TTouch is primarily concerned with stimulating seldom-used neural pathways to the brain. TTouch practitioners also report intriguing success with ear stimulation similar to that mentioned in the discussion of acupuncture. The ears are held between the fingers and stimulated with a stroking motion.

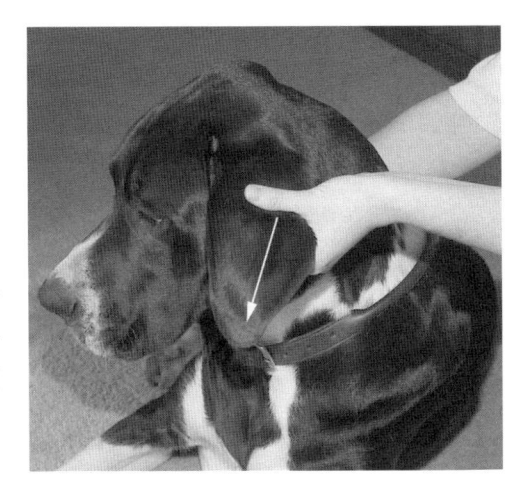

Dog owners can learn and practice TTouch in a number of ways. Books, videos, and workshops offer instruction. Dog owners also have the option of seeking professional treatments performed by certified TTouch practitioners. Practitioners may be located through listings on the Internet or through holistic veterinary clinics.

Herbs

It is best to have a holistic veterinarian guide you in the use of herbs. While many people consider herbs to be a gentler form of treatment, they may have potent interactions with prescription medications. It is important that your veterinarian be aware of all the treatments your dog is receiving.

Medicinal herbs may work best when they are given at intermittent intervals. Your veterinarian may recommend that you give the herb for five days and then skip two days. This pattern may continue for a month or two, followed by a week's rest without any herbs. The cycle may then be repeated.

The following are some herbs that dog owners have found helpful in supporting normal brain function: Black cohosh, valarian, skullcap, oatstraw, and ginko biloba. Frequently, it is possible to find herbs combined in formulas that address a particular problem such as stress or neurological dysfunction. Relax Caps and Calm (see Suppliers section) are two of these. Holistic veterinarians may also recommend Chinese herb formulas or homeopathic treatments such as Silica. (See page 109-110 for information on herbs used for liver support.)

Flower Essence Therapy

Rescue Remedy (also known as Bach Five Flower Essence) is a liquid extract that some owners report beneficial to their dogs. Rescue Remedy contains essence of impatiens, star of Bethlehem, cherry plum, rock rose, and clematis. It is considered safe for use by humans and pets and may be effective in reducing signs of stress, especially postictal pacing and restlessness. Rescue Remedy is available at health food stores, pet supply stores, through holistic veterinarians, or the Internet. Similar products include Stop Stress and Pet Calm.

On average, dog owners give 4 drops of Rescue Remedy to a medium-size dog. For small dogs (under 20 pounds) the recommendation is to give 1 drop for every five pounds of body weight. For large dogs, 4 drops are recommended for the first twenty pounds and then one additional drop for every ten pounds, thereafter. For example, a 90-pound dog might need as many as 11 drops.

Drops may be applied to the gum line or drizzled on top of a spoonful of preservative-free ice cream. (In the United States, Breyer's Ice Cream is a good choice.) Rescue Remedy may also be rubbed on to the ear leather — the hairless area on the inside of the earflap. Owners have varying degrees of success with these products as their dogs are individuals and respond differently.

Physical Exercise

There is a tendency for owners to be overprotective of their epileptic dogs. This may even extend to the elimination of physical activities. This has a major drawback, however, since regular exercise is one of the most effective ways of lowering cortisol levels. Moderate exercise, such as a 20-minute walk, three to four times a week, is highly beneficial for both dog and owner. Water play and swimming should be monitored more closely. If a dog were to seize while swimming, rescue would obviously be more difficult.

Do, however, protect your dog from extreme or prolonged activities. Overexertion, hypoglycemia, and dehydration associated with heavy exercise can precipitate a seizure. Keep a seizure kit with you on long hikes and camping trips. *If* you begin to notice a pattern between periods of heavy exercise and increased seizure frequency, then it may be best to cut back to more moderate levels. Competitive dog sports (obedience, agility, hunting, herding, etc.) include the additional element of psychological stress. This topic will be discussed more fully in Chapter 11, *Additional Health Concerns*.

Chiropractic Treatment

Chiropractic treatment (Veterinary Orthopedic Manipulation) involves the manual adjustment or alignment of the spinal column. Chiropractic treatments performed by qualified veterinary practitioners may relieve pressure on the brain stem and reduce seizure activity stemming from that area. This may be helpful in cases of trauma or abnormalities of the cervical spine.

References

Clemmons, R.M., "Seizure Disorders in Dogs and Cats," http://pawcare.com/rclemmons, January, 2002.

Ferran, R., "Gold Bead Implants," *The Pet Tribune*, an online newsletter of the Ludlam-Dixie Animal Clinic, Miami, Florida, http://www.naturalpetdoc.com/pettribune.htm, November-December, 2000.

Field, T., "Massage therapy," *Medical Clinics of North America*, 86(1): January, 2002.

Levin, C.D., *Dogs, Diet, and Disease: An Owner's Guide to Diabetes Mellitus, Pancreatitis, Cushing's Disease, and More*. Oregon City: Lantern Publications, 2001.

Panzer, R.B., and Chrisman, C.L., "An Auricular Acupuncture Treatment for Idiopathic Canine Epilepsy: A Preliminary Report," *American Journal of Chinese Medicine*, 22(1): 1994.

Schoen, A.M., "Animal Massage: The Touch That Heals," www.drschoen.com/articles_L2_2_.html, October, 2001.

Schoen, A.M., "Seizures in Dogs & Cats: An Integrative Approach with Natural Options," www.drschoen.com/articles_L2_14_.html, October, 2001.

Tellington-Jones, L., *Getting in TTouch With Your Dog*. N. Promfret, Vermont: Trafalgar Square Publishing, 2001.

Wulff-Tilford, M.L., and Tilford, G.L., *Herbs for Pets*. Irvine: Bow Tie Press, 1999.

Chapter 10

Seizures: Before, During, and After

There are numerous ways to assist your epileptic dog when he has a seizure. Prior to that time, there are several things you can do to prepare. The first of these is building a seizure kit.

The Seizure Kit

Collect all the items you typically use during and after a seizure in one place. These may include any of the following items:

>The name, address, and phone number of your local veterinarian *and* the nearest
>>24-hour emergency clinic
>
>Seizure journal
>Rescue Remedy or other herbal formula
>Rectal thermometer and lubricant (Vaseline, K-Y jelly, etc.)
>Rubbing alcohol
>Small packets of pancake syrup or a small bottle of Karo syrup
>Towels and a spray bottle with a vinegar and water solution to clean-up accidents
>Rectal Valium supplies: Syringe, needle, rectal catheter, and lubricant
>A simple checklist list to keep you focused on your jobs, such as:
>>*Note the time when the seizure starts*
>>Protect dog from injury
>>Turn off appliances
>>Dim the lights
>>Loosen collar if appropriate
>>Confine aggressive pack members
>>*Note the time when the seizure ends*
>>Administer a snack, Rescue Remedy, Valium, or other AEDs, if appropriate

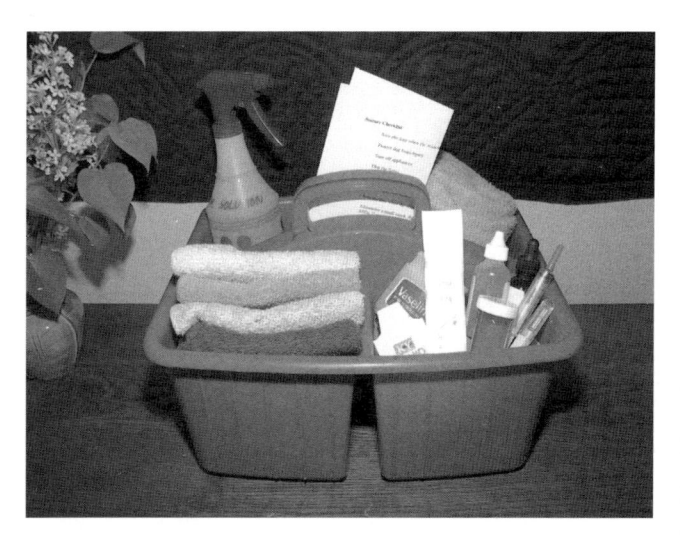

These supplies should be kept at a central location in your house. Store everything in a tray or carry case so that it can all be transported to the dog. If you travel frequently with your dog keep a second seizure kit in the car. Be sure to restock your seizure kit after each use.

In addition, designate a specific spot **in the freezer** for storing preservative-free vanilla ice cream and cooler packs. Remind family members that these are *for the dog*.

In addition to building a seizure kit, you might find it beneficial to outfit your dog with a personalized collar tag that states his epileptic condition and the phone number of your veterinary clinic. Also, plan and practice how you would load a large or unconscious dog into the car should you need to take him to the veterinary clinic.

The Phases of a Seizure

Preictal Phase

The preictal phase is the period that precedes the actual seizure. You may also hear it referred to as the **prodromal period** or **aura**. It is during this period that an epileptic may recognize that a seizure is imminent. It can be helpful for dog owners to become familiar with preictal behaviors. Owners can use these signs to prepare for the onset of — or possibly prevent — the seizure.

Some dogs begin their preictal behaviors early on the day of the seizure. These commonly include **clingy behaviors**. Epileptic dogs may engage in unusual eye contact with their owner, sit close, or follow him from room to room. Some behaviors suggest that the dog is anxious to escape his environment. He may try to hide under furniture.

Other dogs drink excessively or lick or gnaw on their paws prior to a seizure. They may stand on their hind legs, crawl on their bellies, or run back and forth in short bursts. If you suspect your dog may hurt himself on surrounding objects, try to straddle him with your feet or knees in order to keep him safe. Be certain to include both the epileptic's preictal behavior, as well as the behaviors of companion dogs, in your seizure journal. These notes may help you identify subtle patterns.

Seizure Alert Dogs

Dogs can be trained to provide a number of important services. They can be trained as guide dogs for the blind and hearing dogs for the deaf. Nationally recognized instructor, Dawn Jecs, realized that dogs can also be trained to detect imminent seizure activity.

Jecs directed the training of the first-ever seizure alert dog, a role in which the dog signals his human companion that a seizure is about to happen. With this help, a human epileptic can get himself into a safe situation before the seizure occurs. Jecs believes that the remarkable canine sense of smell is responsible for this feat. She and other experts suspect that tremendous neurochemical activity produces an odor detectable only by dogs.

If you have more than one dog, it is possible to implement a similar type of warning system in your own household. In other words, you may be able to train one of your other dogs to alert for the epileptic dog. While researchers at the University of Florida indicate that the *best* seizure alert dogs are those that are attentive and have a close bond to the epileptic, it is possible to train almost all dogs for this function. Some dogs may just be more reliable than others.

In fact, some dogs exhibit this skill naturally. They may try to alert you by pawing, jumping, or making unusual eye contact. Some dogs bark wildly or make strange vocalizations. Others lie down close to the epileptic dog, close to their owner, or begin to circle and pace. Such warnings may come hours, minutes, or more often, just a few seconds before the seizure.

If your dog naturally exhibits these behaviors reward him with verbal praise such as, "That's a very, good dog!" and offer him a food treat. Rewards will increase the likelihood that these behaviors will be repeated. If the dog does not alert you naturally, it is possible for you to teach him how.

To train a seizure alert dog you will first need to identify a skill that will become his alerting behavior. For example, this could involve placing a paw on your leg, lying down in front of you, or even jumping up in the air. Choose a behavior that suits your dog's temperament and one that he does not associate with another meaning.

Do some preliminary training apart from the time of an actual seizure. This need only take a moment or two each day. Evening television time is usually sufficient.

Prepare some training treats before you begin. Small pieces of chicken work well.

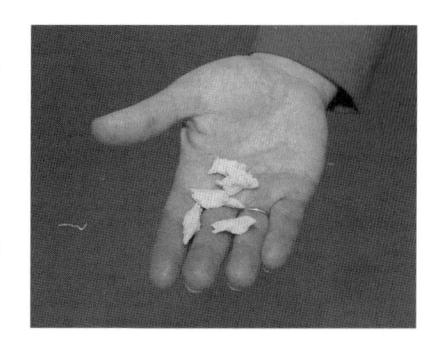

If you wish to train a behavior such as pawing your leg, lift the dog's paw onto your leg or foot and feed him a treat. Alternately, you can press down on his paw, which will likely cause him to lift it up. Quickly slide your foot under his so he will step on you as he puts his paw down.

Many instructors believe that dogs learn faster when they perform an activity on their own. As you repeat the exercise, the dog may place his paw on your leg by himself. Tell him how smart he is! Offer him a "jackpot" of treats — three, four, or five treats in succession. This will make a greater impression upon him. Some dogs are very slow to make the connection. Don't lose patience. It may take several weeks or even a month to learn the new skill.

Once the dog is reliably placing his paw on your leg give the behavior a name, such as "paw." The next step is to use this training in conjunction with an actual seizure. This step is, admittedly, a little trickier. Since attending to the epileptic dog should be your first priority, training an alert dog may best be done with the help of a family member or after the seizure has stopped.

If you can enlist the help of a family member, agree ahead of time who will attend to the seizing dog and who will train the alert dog. When either of you recognizes the beginning of a seizure, call the other to work. As the seizure begins ask the alert dog for his behavior. If he offers his paw, reward him heavily. If he does not, view it as another training opportunity. Place his paw on your leg and then reward him.

If you are without an assistant, ask the alert dog for the behavior *after the seizure* has concluded. The biochemical odor of the seizure may still be present. Reward the alert dog lavishly while the epileptic recovers.

With a multifaceted treatment program, your epileptic dog may not experience many seizures. When he does, alerting behaviors can be beneficial. Such warning may help you protect the dog from injury or give you time to interrupt the seizure.

Arresting Behaviors

Long before medications became available to control epilepsy, ancient people practiced other methods of naturally halting or minimizing seizure activity. These methods are still recommended today. You may hear them described as methods of "naturally arresting" seizures or methods of "sensory arrest."

Sensory arrest involves stimulating the area of the brain that is threatened with electrical discharge. This can be accomplished with a strong sound, physical touch, or taste. It is suspected that by giving these neurons a strong stimulus, the random discharge of seizure activity can be overridden. When the patient's attention shifts from the inward focus to an outward focus (the new stimulus) it seems to help enforce the inhibitory response of the surrounding neurons.

Sensory arrest is most successful when patients have a highly identifiable aura. In reviewing your journal notes you may be able to identify behaviors that indicate your dog's aura or preictal phase. When an owner recognizes the onset of this aura, stimulus can be applied in an attempt to thwart the impending seizure.

Learning effective arresting behaviors is an individualized matter. One method, called "**startle and shake**," is taught by a number of human neurologists with success. This method involves holding the patient by the shoulders, shaking him firmly once or twice, and saying, "No!" or "Stop!"

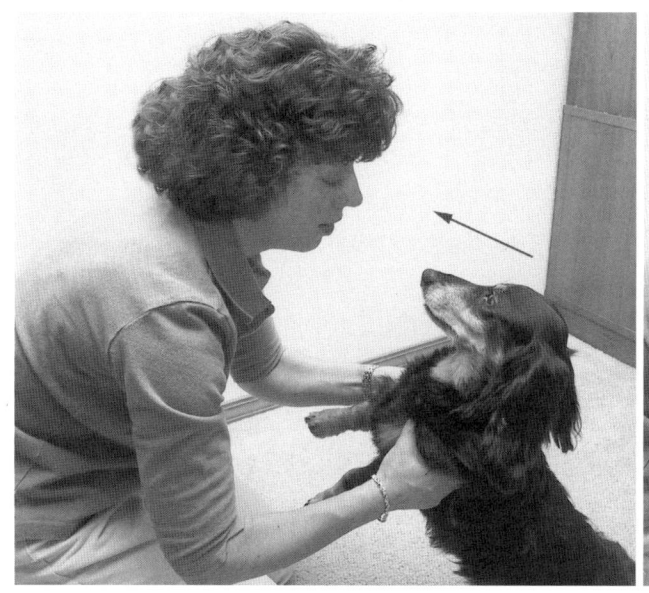

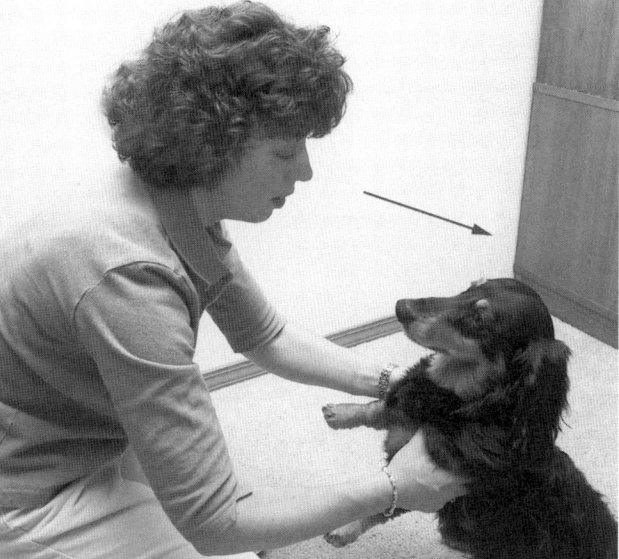

Touch can be an effective way to arrest seizures. One mother found tickling stopped her son's seizures. For humans who experience "tingling" seizures, getting up, moving around, and slapping their arms and legs has proven successful. Try vigorously stroking or patting your dog's neck and back.

In **acupuncture** theory, there is a slight depression on the top of the dog's head known as the GV20 point. This area is considered to be a pressure point that will encourage general sedation. Some dog owners have reported successfully arresting seizures by gently rubbing this area. Two points located on the ears, named Shen Men 1 and Shen Men 2, have also been reported effective in reducing the extent and frequency of seizures.

If your dog has a tremor in an extremity it may be helpful to apply **ligature pressure** above that area with your hand. This particular method of seizure arrest in humans dates back to ancient Greek times.

Some dog owners report success by applying a **cold pack** to the dog's head or to the part of the body that is typically involved in the seizure. This can be as simple as a cool, wet washcloth, or the type of cooler pack that remains in the freezer until needed. Wrap the latter inside a cloth before applying.

Some owners and veterinarians practice **ocular compression**. This involves *slight* finger pressure against the lids with the eyes closed for ten to 60 seconds. This is suspected to stimulate the vagus nerve, a cranial nerve that runs down from the brain, through the face, neck, and thorax (chest cavity), to the abdomen. Stimulation of the vagus nerve is thought to interrupt impending electrical discharge in areas of the brain that are prone to seizures. (Do not practice ocular compression if your dog is suspected to have eye problems.)

Scents and **flavors** may also be able to arrest seizures. Some parents are able to arrest their children's absence seizures with the strong scent of jasmine. The sense of taste has been successfully used, too. Some owners report good results offering Rescue Remedy drizzled on a spoonful of preservative-free ice cream or rubbed into the ear leather.

Finally, dogs can be distracted from an impending seizure by initiating **physical activity**. This may include calling the dog to you, throwing a ball for him, or suggesting that you "go for a walk." Simply getting the dog to open his mouth for a treat or a toy can arrest partial seizures (head tremors) in some dogs.

Physical activity may also be helpful in disrupting preictal paw-licking behaviors. Try to distract the dog with another activity or offer him something to eat. Try various treats during the preictal phase. Keep a log of what you've tried and which methods, if any, work.

> Important note:
> *Do not attempt arresting tactics once the aura has progressed into a full-blown, generalized seizure.*

Ictal Phase

The ictal phase refers to the period of actual seizure activity. It usually lasts for only **one to two minutes**. Typical behaviors of a generalized seizure may include: Loss of consciousness and an increase in motor activity such as spasms, stiffening, jerking, head-shaking, running motion of the legs, rapid clamping and foaming of the mouth, or loss of bowel, bladder, or anal gland control. This massive neural and physical activity releases hormones such as prolactin, ACTH, and cortisol. Large amounts of glucose are also consumed during this time.

According to human epileptics, seizures themselves do not hurt. This can be difficult to believe during the chilling howling some dogs emit. Experts believe this is merely air vibrating past their vocal cords.

The ictal phase of a *partial* seizure may include a change in consciousness or "blanking out." It may include a tremor of a certain body part, hallucinations, or changes in mood and behavior.

What To Do During a Seizure

Take a deep breath. *Note the time when the seizure starts*. Turn off vacuum, radio, or television noise. Have family members speak softly. Dim the lights. Get your seizure kit and checklist. A checklist may help you stay focused at this highly emotional moment.

Keep the dog from injuring himself. This may involve helping him to the ground or even catching him if he is about to fall. If your dog has collapsed into pillows or bedding in such a way that impairs breathing, gently reposition the bedding or his head. Prevent him from scratching himself in the face if he is inclined to do so. Sometimes it is best to attend to the dog first and then secure your seizure kit, dim the lights, etc., after the seizure. If other family members can assist you, it may be possible to do these things simultaneously.

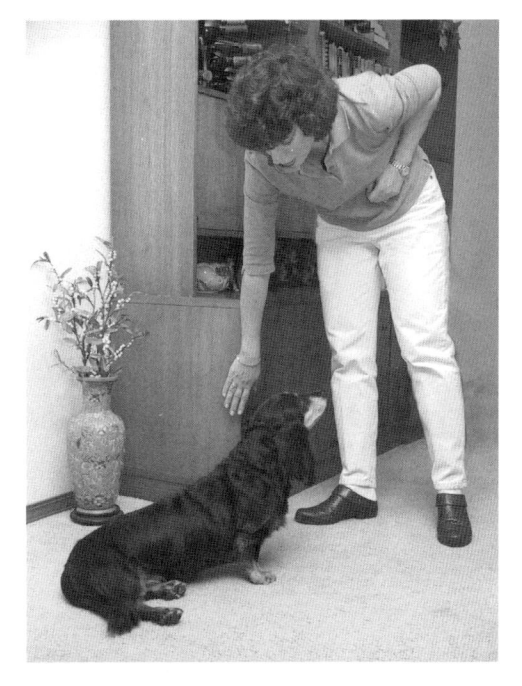

If your dog typically stays on his feet, crawls, or continues to move around, remain close to him. Try to position yourself between the dog and any furniture he might hit. If he is on the bed or couch when the seizure begins prevent him from falling off the furniture.

Do not attempt to place anything in the dog's mouth. This is especially true if he is actively snapping his jaws. It is rare, if not impossible, for a dog to "swallow his tongue" but the risk of incurring a severe bite wound is very real. *Be sure to note the time when the seizure ends.*

Pack Members' Behaviors

Pack members may demonstrate a variety of behaviors when the epileptic dog seizes. As indicated, some pack members may offer alerting behaviors to either you or the seizure dog.

Once the ictal phase has started, some pack members will simply watch from a distance or even hide from the activity. Others may try to lick the seizing dog. A few dogs seem confused by the seizure and revert to "survival of the fittest" instincts. These dogs may mount or **attack the seizing dog**.

Yet other dogs may fight amongst *themselves* while the epileptic seizes. Obviously, it is best to separate these dogs at the onset of a seizure. If these problems are serious at your house and seizures are frequent, consider separating such dogs when you leave the house or retire for the evening.

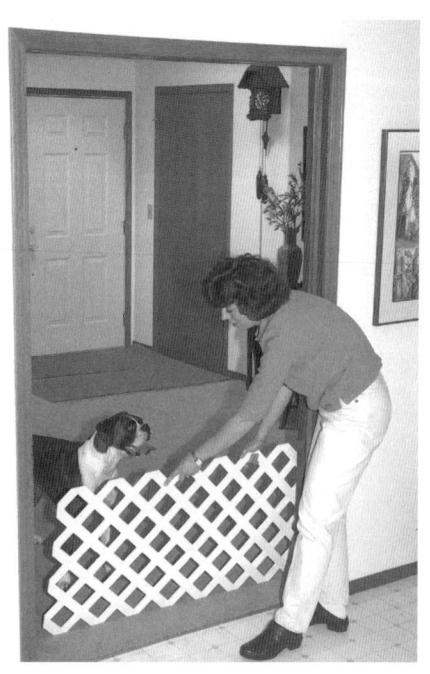

Postictal Phase

The postictal phase is the period following the seizure that may last between a few minutes and several hours. Some dogs "are not themselves" for as long as a day or more.

Following a seizure, levels of ACTH, cortisol, and other stress-related hormones rise significantly. Symptoms of excess cortisol include: Heat intolerance, ravenous appetite, excess thirst, confusion (getting stuck in a corner, hiding behind furniture, howling, or barking), and mood changes (aggression, depression, restlessness, pacing, or prowling). Such behaviors commonly last for 30 minutes or more. These dogs appear to be unaware of their actions. Some dogs may experience temporary blindness.

Human epilepsy patients report common postictal feelings of confusion, headache, and fatigue. While muscles may be slightly sore, humans do not report a memory of the seizure being painful.

What To Do After a Seizure

Many owners offer their dog a **small snack** directly after a seizure. The snack can consist of a spoonful of pancake syrup or *preservative-free* vanilla ice cream (such as the Breyer's brand). This can help replace blood sugar consumed during the seizure. Once the dog is back to normal, offer him a larger snack. Certain dogs may *not* be interested in food until they have fully recovered.

Owners often top the ice cream with a few drops of Rescue Remedy or other **herbal supplement**. In some cases this appears to minimize the restless behaviors and help calm the dog.

If your dog has generalized *cluster* seizures, it may also be helpful to administer an extra dose of his antiepileptic medication (such as Pb or KBr) after the dog is alert enough to safely swallow. Discuss this option with your veterinarian. This is also the time to administer the **rectal Valium** procedure if it has been prescribed for your dog. (See page 82 for details.) Some veterinarians also prescribe *oral* Valium as part of this protocol.

If your dog is **restless** after the seizure, try to reduce cortisol levels by performing massage. It is possible that administering the dietary supplement Phosphatidyl Serine will also reduce cortisol levels but it may take several hours to become effective.

Keep your dog safe during the postictal phase. Many dogs are **disoriented** and unsteady on their feet, yet, they may still try to get up and follow their owners about the house. An exercise pen (ex-pen) placed around the dog will help keep him safe, as will a baby gate or other blockade at the top of the staircase. Some dogs have a need to reintroduce themselves to the pack following a seizure. This can include human family members as well as other dogs and even cats.

Seizure activity, and cortisol release, may activate very primal behaviors in some dogs. These dogs sense they are incapacitated and vulnerable and may protect themselves with **aggressive behavior**. Normally placid dogs may snap and growl at family members. Respect the dog's space until he has completely recovered. Pretend you are unconcerned. Speak to him calmly and gently from a short distance. These dogs will usually rise and return to their owners when *they* are ready for contact.

When generalized seizures occur close together they can have the effect of raising **body temperature**. Take a rectal temperature reading if your dog experiences cluster seizures. A reading greater than 107 F (or 41.5 C) can be dangerous and requires veterinary care.

Designate one thermometer in the house, as the dog's thermometer. Keep it in your seizure kit. To **take a rectal temperature**, first shake down the thermometer until the mercury level reads 96 F or so. Lubricate the tip of the thermometer with Vaseline or K-Y jelly. Lift the dog's tail. With a twisting motion, insert the thermometer to a depth of one or two inches (slightly less for small dogs and slightly more for large dogs). Stop if you feel resistance. The thermometer must be deep enough to register true rectal temperature but not so deep as to cause discomfort. Keep the thermometer inserted for about a minute. After reading the thermometer wipe it clean with rubbing alcohol.

The normal range for canine rectal temperature is between 100 F and 102.5 F (or 37.5 C and 40 C). If your dog's temperature is elevated, attempt to cool him. If his temperature exceeds 107 F (or 41.5 C), take your dog to the veterinary clinic.

Lowering body temperature may help interrupt the cluster activity and prevent organ damage. Carry the dog to a cooler room or safe outdoor area. Do *not* wrap a dog in towels or cover him in ice. Instead, wet down areas from which the dog can lose heat such as the throat, chest, underbelly, and inner thighs. Some owners wrap freezer packs inside towels for this use. Some wipe the footpads with rubbing alcohol.

Allow the dog to rest after a seizure. You too, may find this to be a good time to regroup. Canine seizures can be psychologically exhausting for owners, as well as dogs. Reorganize your seizure kit. Call your veterinarian to refill any medications that are running low.

Document the Seizure Activity in Your Journal:

> The start time and date of the seizure
> The dog's location (room, car, public park, etc.) during the seizure
> What activities or incidents preceded the seizure (exercise, vacuuming, etc.)
> Pre-seizure behaviors (pacing, licking, unusual eye contact, and the length of time they occurred prior to the seizure)
> A description of the seizure (type, severity, loss of bladder control, length of duration, etc.)
> Post-seizure behaviors (type and duration)
> Include both the dog's behaviors and yours, such as medications or supplements you gave after the seizure and any arresting techniques that you believe successfully stopped or minimized the seizure

Bring Your Dog to the Veterinary Clinic When:

> Your dog does not recover between two seizures
> The seizure appears to last longer than three or four minutes
> Your dog has multiple seizures within a one-hour period
> He is not breathing or is having difficulty breathing
> He injures himself during the seizure
> His temperature exceeds 107 F (or 41.5 C)

If possible, call the clinic to let them know that you are bringing in your dog. Take your seizure journal, seizure kit, and the name and phone number of your regular veterinarian with you. (The latter applies if you are going to a 24-hour emergency clinic where they do not know your dog's history.)

The following are some suggestions for owners that must lift a large, unconscious, or **groggy dog into the car**. Try wrapping a towel under his belly as a sling. Improvise a ramp with sturdy lumber. Brace the bottom so the top of the ramp does not slip out of the car. Duct tape might work for this. If you can roll the dog onto a towel or drop cloth, it may be possible to slide him up the ramp. If there are neighbors on the street, don't be shy. Call out, "I need help!" While none of these options are optimum, they may help you get your dog to the clinic in time for life-saving veterinary attention.

References

Carlson, D.G., and Giffin, J.M., *Dog Owner's Home Veterinary Handbook*. New York: Howell Book House, 1992.

Mark, J.M., "Seizure Alert Dogs," http://www.vetcentric.com/magazine/magazineArticle.cfm?ARTICLEID=1456, April, 2000.

Maun, K., "When Your Dog Has Seizures — Coping With a Scary Situation," *Dog Nose News*, 2(3): October, 2001.

Oliver, J.E., Lorenz, M.D., and Kornegay, J.N., *Handbook of Veterinary Neurology, Third Edition*. Philadelphia: WB Saunders Company, 1997.

Richard, A., and Reiter, J., *Epilepsy: A New Approach*. New York: Prentice Hall, 1990.

Speciale, J., and Stahlbrodt, J.E., "Use of Ocular Compression to Induce Vagal Stimulation and Aid in Controlling Seizures in Seven Dogs," *Journal of the American Veterinary Medical Association*, 214(5): 1999.

Wulff-Tilford, M.L., and Tilford, G.L., *Herbs for Pets*. Irvine: Bow Tie Press, 1999.

Chapter 11

Additional Health Concerns

There are a number of additional health concerns that may affect your dog. Some are the result of high cortisol levels, some are related to the dog's compromised immune system, and others are a result of the high levels of chemicals present in daily life. Health problems frequently occur in combination since the dog's entire immune/digestive/endocrine system is stressed.

In many cases, prevention is the best medicine. You may not be able to forestall every health problem, but catching them in their early stages can be beneficial for your dog. The first step in this process is to perform frequent physical assessments. This involves a head-to-toe examination of your dog to check for signs of infection, injury, or changes in his skin or coat. Such an examination can also be combined with therapeutic massage — an excellent way to help reduce the effects of stress.

Preventive Health Measures

Physical Assessment

Begin by examining your dog's head. Look inside his ears, mouth, and at his teeth and gums. Signs of infection can include swelling, unpleasant odor, or discharge. Examine his eyes. Check for cloudiness or discharge. Gently lift the upper eyelid and check that the "whites of his eyes" are white, not red.

Run your hands over his head, through his fur, and down his neck. Check for any injuries, lacerations, bumps, and lumps. Run your hands along his back, his chest, and each side of his body. Check each leg and the pads of his feet. Gently spread apart his toes. Check for irritation (redness) or yeasty skin infection (often accompanied by redness or brown discharge). Check between your dog's hind legs and around his tail. The skin fold between the thighs is a common location for skin irritations to develop. Urinary tract infections can cause redness, swelling, discharge, and dribbling urine.

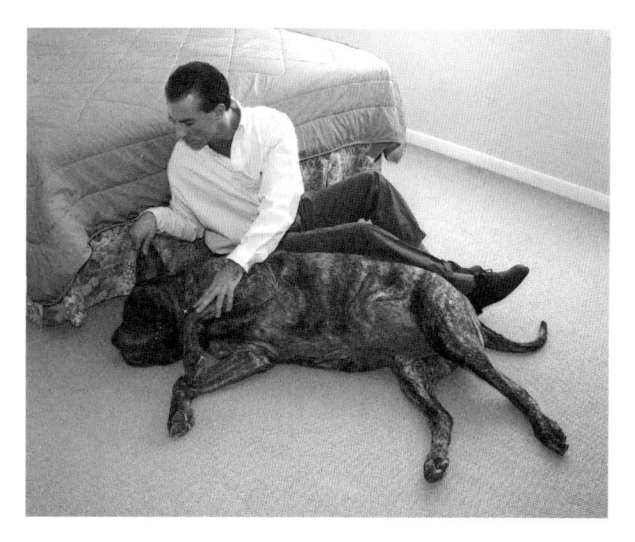

Complete an assessment several times each week. Choose a time when the dog is relaxed. It is a pleasurable activity for most dogs and their owners, and can easily be combined with massage therapy, TTouch, or acupressure. (See Chapter 9, *Alternative Therapies*.) Report changes or unusual findings to your veterinarian.

Other Preventive Measures

If your dog continues to experience frequent infections, incontinence, or gastrointestinal problems, try switching your dog to a homemade diet, if you have not already done so. It may not eliminate all complications, but it may help reduce the frequency and severity of symptoms.

Infections

Several factors contribute to the high incidence of infections in chronically ill dogs. Depressed immune system function (white blood cell activity) and a high-sugar environment (conducive to bacterial growth) are two of these. Yeast is a common cause of infections. It, too, thrives on excess sugar and reproduces quickly in moist conditions. Some dog owners describe the dark-brown discharge of yeast infection as "the creeping crud."

Infections can result in a vicious cycle. They raise blood glucose levels. Higher blood glucose levels demand a greater production of insulin. This cycle further exhausts the beta cells of the pancreas. Chronic infection causes the release of cortisol as part of the immune system response. This, too, results in high blood sugar and greater chance for infection. If prescription steroids have been prescribed, they will also contribute to this cycle.

In most cases of infection, oral antibiotics will be prescribed for your dog. It is crucial that your dog complete the entire course of medication, even if symptoms appear to subside. If a dog is only medicated for a few days, the bacteria can become *stronger* and more resistant to drug treatment in the future. Antibiotics may be prescribed for a few weeks, a month, or even longer periods in severe cases.

If your veterinarian does prescribe antibiotics, consider adding the beneficial bacteria, lactobacillus acidophilus — available in yogurt or powder form — to your dog's diet. Antibiotics kill beneficial bacteria in the intestine and adding acidophilus prevents the overgrowth of more aggressive bacteria. You may also find specific preparations known as probiotic powders. These include a combination of several beneficial bacteria and are available from veterinarians or pet supply stores. (See Suppliers section.)

Skin Infections

Yeast and fungal growth can occur between toes, around the face, and at the ends of long ears. If in doubt, your veterinarian can do a skin scraping to diagnose the problem. Common signs of skin infection include itching, licking (especially of the paws), a dark greasy discharge, and possible hair loss.

Help prevent yeast infections by minimizing damp environments. Be sure to dry off wet feet when the dog comes in from the rain or snow. Clip long hair around feet so they dry faster. Wipe beards and faces dry after a drink in the water bowl. Purchase special bowls (tall, thin, and bucket-shaped) to keep long ears from getting wet. (See Suppliers section.)

Apply an antifungal powder (often available from your veterinarian or over the counter at your local pharmacy) in between toes and skin folds. Your veterinarian will likely prescribe oral or topical antibiotics and possibly a medicated shampoo, as well.

Ear Infections

Yeast and bacteria growth inside the ears can produce a dark greasy discharge with an unpleasant odor. Common signs include scratching and head-shaking behaviors. Occasionally, infection and scarring can cause deafness or equilibrium problems.

It is important to keep the ear canal clean. Your veterinarian may prescribe a cleansing and drying solution to use inside the ears, as well as oral antibiotics and topical steroids. These infections can be very tenacious and difficult to cure.

Urinary Tract Infections (UTIs)

UTIs can involve several structures, including the kidneys, but most often refer to infections of the bladder. Several factors contribute to bladder infections. These can include glucosuria (glucose in the urine), depressed white blood cell function, immunoglobulin A (IgA) deficiency, and the high levels of impurities (chemicals and poor-quality protein) present in commercial diets. The latter irritate and inflame the bladder lining much as they inflame the intestinal lining. This inflammation primes the bladder for infection.

Signs of UTIs can include frequent licking of the urethra, incontinence or dribbling of urine, blood in the urine, straining, urgency (frequently asking to go outside) without being able to produce much volume, increased thirst, and lethargy.

To diagnose a bladder infection, your veterinarian may request that you collect a urine sample and deliver it to the clinic. There are several ways to do this. The urine sample does not need to be sterile for this examination, only clean. You can use a clean ceramic mug, margarine container, or plastic zip-style bag.

Follow the dog into the yard. Walk along with him, but pretend you are not very interested in his activities. Most dogs are accustomed to relieving themselves, *by* themselves, and may be intimidated if their owner follows them. After the dog squats or lifts his leg, quietly slip the cup or container under the urine stream once he has started. If he seems especially alarmed by what you are doing, offer him a food treat afterward.

If your aim is poor and the idea of urine on your hand bothers you, purchase a pair or box of latex gloves. You may also use a clean pooper-scooper or soup ladle to catch the urine, transferring it to a small container afterward. This alleviates the need to bend down.

It is best to bring a fresh urine sample (within an hour of collection) to your veterinarian. If this is not possible, refrigerate the urine sample until it is time to leave for the clinic. This will help prevent excess bacteria from growing in the sample and skewing the findings.

In more difficult UTI cases, your veterinarian may obtain a sterile sample by performing a bladder tap. Urine is collected through a sterile needle inserted through the skin, directly into the bladder. This can provide a more accurate urine sample when there is difficulty identifying or treating infectious agents.

Your veterinarian may encourage you to add acidic fruit or supplements to your dog's diet: Cranberries, blueberries, cranberry supplement, or Azocran tablets. All of these acidify the urine, which helps to discourage bacterial growth. You can monitor urine acidity with pH urine test strips, available at your local pharmacy.

Dietary Management of Infection

Canine nutritionists recommend treating chronic infections from the inside of the body, outward. In addition to the treatments your veterinarian prescribes, nutritionists recommend acidifying the dog's system through dietary means. If you are feeding a homemade food, remove any grain and high-sugar fruits and vegetables from the diet. This includes bananas, apples, sweet potatoes, yams, carrots, green peas, corn, parsnips, winter squash, and tomatoes.

Commercial dog food, especially kibble, is very alkaline. If you continue to feed commercial food, acidify the system by adding vitamin C, *raw* apple cider vinegar (available at health food stores, not grocery stores), cranberry juice, cranberry extract, or frozen blueberries. In addition, some research indicates that *highly bio-available protein* (homemade diets with raw *or* cooked meat) discourages bacteria from developing in the urinary tract.

Renal (Kidney) Problems

Kidney Infection

Frequent or long-term, low-grade bladder infections can travel into the kidneys. Signs of kidney infection can include dilute urine, blood in the urine, vomiting, and decreased appetite. These, like bladder infections, are treated with potent, sometimes long-term antibiotics.

Kidney Degeneration

Apart from kidney *infection*, is the problem of kidney *degeneration*: The gradual loss of kidney function. Signs can include dilute urine, dehydration, and electrolyte imbalance. Chronic kidney degeneration can also result in anemia, weakness, and loss of appetite.

Kidneys that are scarred from dietary impurities and function poorly cannot filter excess phosphorus or uremic acids from the bloodstream. When phosphorus accumulates, the body pulls calcium from the bones to bind the phosphorus and carry it away. This is another way in which high levels of calcium accumulates in the blood stream and soft tissues of the body. Clinical signs can include joint pain, lameness, and itchiness. When uremic acids accumulate they can contribute to seizures.

Two schools of thought exist as to how best to deal with kidney disease. Most veterinarians prescribe specially formulated, low-protein, low-phosphorous commercial diets. They believe these will minimize uremic toxins and slow down renal failure. Advanced cases may require intravenous or subcutaneous fluid and electrolyte replacement at the veterinary clinic.

Other experts recommend feeding a home-prepared diet consisting of moderate amounts (50% or less) of high-quality, biologically appropriate protein. This includes fish, eggs, chicken, beef, or lamb. If possible, you may wish to alternate meals of mostly protein, with meals that are mostly vegetables. This allows the kidneys to rest during the low protein meals.

Incontinence

Steroid-induced Incontinence

Cortisol, cortisone drugs, and some AEDs have similar, steroid-like effects. They break down muscle tissue (catabolism), causing muscle weakness and wasting. This effect is not limited to skeletal muscles. Cortisol and steroid-like medications can weaken bladder wall and sphincter muscles, causing urinary incontinence and dribbling. Reducing cortisol production can be an effective means of minimizing incontinence.

Treating Incontinence

There are several ways you can reduce the nuisance and number of urinary accidents around the house. Some methods involve behavior modification and dietary management. Others include physical aids and items that make living with chronic incontinence less troublesome.

Behavioral Issues and Incontinence

When you are home, pay attention to your dog's schedule, his water intake, and his body language. Some dogs are better than others about "asking" to go out. They will make eye contact with you, wander near the door, or whine. Other dogs never ask. The owners of these dogs must pay attention to the clock (when was the last time the dog went out?) and water consumption and encourage the dog to go again. Dogs typically need to urinate after activity (play) and, often, after napping.

Have a specific word or phrase for elimination. There are times when it is helpful to have a dog eliminate upon command. Some owners say, "Do your business" or "Potty." You can help add this word to his vocabulary by saying, "good business" or "good potty," after he's done and by rewarding with a food treat. Keep treats handy by the back door.

If your dog does have an accident, do not carry on about it. Calmly help the dog out the door and say whatever phrase you use for him to eliminate, reminding him that the outdoors is the appropriate place for this. In most cases, however, these are not lapses in house training but rather, *uncontrollable* accidents.

Yelling or spanking can make a dog quite nervous about eliminating. A nervous dog is even less likely to ask to go out. You can clean up the accident while the dog is outdoors.

Cleaning Up Accidents

Deodorizing the spot reduces the chances of another accident happening in the same area. One of the oldest and best remedies is white vinegar. For urine accidents on carpet, repeatedly blot up the area. Lean your weight against small piles of towels until no more is absorbed.

Saturate the area with a solution of half water and half vinegar and cover it with a towel so that dirt is not tracked through the area. If the spot smells of anything other than the faint fragrance of vinegar after a day or two, repeat the process.

Dietary Issues and Incontinence

A number of dog owners report that dietary changes affect canine incontinence. They contend that eliminating grains from their dog's diet improves bladder control. This may be linked to the cycle of inflammation, cortisol production, and muscle weakness that grain protein is believed to induce.

Mechanical Aids and Items for Incontinence

If the accidents are frequent, consider making some concessions for your dog. If you do not have a doggy door to the yard, consider installing one. Consider purchasing housebreaking pads. These are a combination of absorbent paper toweling with a plastic backing. They are often scented so that puppies are attracted to eliminate on them. Similar pads are available in pharmacies or hospital supply stores for incontinent humans. These pads are larger in size than the puppy pads. If an older dog has repeated accidents in the same spot, you can put the pads there to protect that particular area in your house.

If there is a place in the house, garage, laundry room, etc., where you would be willing to let the dog relieve himself, put the pads there. Since most dogs do not like eliminating in the house once they have been housebroken, you may have to let your dog know that this spot is now acceptable to you.

Lead him to the spot at a time he normally eliminates, give him the command to eliminate — even if it is something such as, "Do you want to go out?" Tap the paper pads and give him a food treat if he eliminates. You may even scent the pads with a few drops of his urine if you collect it for laboratory tests.

The owner of one large, geriatric dog was unable to make it home from work each day, before her dog needed to relieve himself. She set up a child's rigid, plastic swimming pool (the type that is about 8 to 10 inches high), lined it with newspapers, and placed it in her basement. Litter boxes designed specifically for dogs are available at some larger pet supply stores.

One owner, whose dog slept in another room of the house, purchased a baby monitor. With one monitor by the dog's bed, and one by hers, she was able to hear when the dog needed to go out at night.

Another owner purchased the type of rigid plastic carpet protector that fits underneath rolling desk chairs. In this way, she was able to hear the dog's toenails tap if the dog got out of bed during the night. The plastic served the dual purpose of preventing accidents in the dog's bed from leaking down onto the carpeting below. Plastic drop clothes and plastic-lined mattress pads can serve the same purpose. Mattress pads can also be used to cover favorite furniture.

Some people move the dog's sleeping quarters into a tiled or vinyl-floored bathroom. And there are certain dog beds available that will allow urine to pass through webbed bedding to a pan below. (See Suppliers section.)

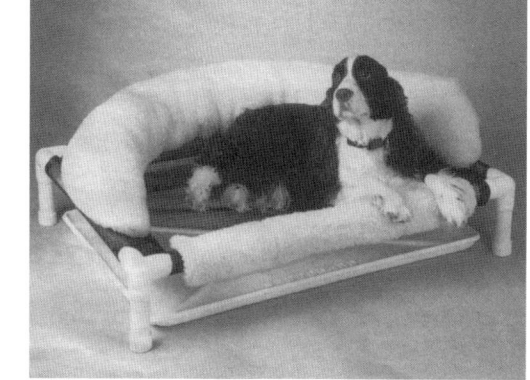

Photo courtesy of SleePee-Time Beds

Some owners purchase or construct doggy diapers for incontinent pets. To diaper a male dog, purchase a regular diaper for human infants and several elastic dress clips, the type used to gather the fabric on the back of a dress. These are sold in fabric and fashion accessory stores. You can find similar elasticized clips designed to hold sheets on the bed in the bed linen department. Apply the diaper like a cummerbund. Line the diaper with feminine sanitary pads for additional absorbency. Diapers for female dogs are available commercially.

While some of these measures may seem extravagant, both dog and owner can benefit from them. Creating a situation where your dog can continue to be a clean and tidy pet improves the quality of his life, and probably yours, as well.

Hepatic (Liver) Disease

The liver is involved in nearly all aspects of metabolism so liver disease, regardless of cause, will affect almost every system in the body. The excessive chemical additives found in commercial diets chronically irritate and strain the liver. This strain impairs the liver's ability to filter out debris and process food molecules in the bloodstream.

Once the body begins reacting to chronic inflammation (bowel, pancreas, and bladder), the liver must also filter out high levels of circulating hormones, such as adrenal estrogen and cortisol. Long-term cortisol (or prescription cortisone) can cause lesions to develop on the liver. The addition of antiepileptic drugs (AEDs) causes even greater strain and damage.

Signs of liver disease may include any of the following: Loss of appetite, vomiting, diarrhea, weight loss, the appearance of abdominal pain or swollen abdomen, jaundice, (yellow pigment seen in the "whites" of the eyes) increased water consumption, or lethargy.

Your veterinarian may recommend one of many diagnostic measures to accurately diagnose your dog's liver problems. Blood work will evaluate blood cell counts and possible anemia. Blood chemistry analysis will examine the function of the liver as it attempts to process glucose, bilirubin, and urea. It will also evaluate electrolyte levels, albumin, globulin, and bile acid levels. The following values are typically elevated in liver disease: Enzymes such as alkaline phosphatase (ALKP), alanine aminotransferase (ALT), and bilirubin. Other values, such as albumin, protein, and blood urea nitrogen (BUN) are typically low. Additionally, your veterinarian may wish to run a urine analysis, radiographs/x-rays, ultrasound, or a liver biopsy.

Measuring bile acid levels is considered one of the best tests available for evaluating liver function. Since little, if any, bile should escape the portal system (circulation between the liver, gallbladder, and intestine), any leakage into general circulation is considered a sign of liver dysfunction.

The bile acid test consists of drawing a blood sample following a period of fasting, usually 12 hours. The dog is then fed a fairly high-calorie meal. Two hours later, a second blood sample is collected. The after-meal (or postprandial) sample will normally be somewhat higher than the first sample, but both should be within the normal range indicated by the laboratory (typically, less than 20 umol/L).

Since the liver can regenerate itself, it is especially valuable to reduce the irritants that cause liver damage. Again, consider switching to a homemade diet without grains, if you have not already done so. Liver lesions caused by high levels of cortisol *are* reversible, although it may take several months time. (See pages 109-110 for dietary supplements commonly recommended for liver support.)

Hypothyroidism: Diagnoses and Treatment

This section discusses testing modes and treatment methods. (For a detailed discussion of the causes of thyroid disease, see Chapter 5, *Seizure-provoking Factors*.)

Thyroid Testing

There are numerous tests available for evaluating thyroid function. These tests are continually being updated and improved. Typically, doctors have relied upon a measurement of T4 levels to diagnose thyroid disease. This thyroid test is commonly performed in veterinary medicine. However, this test alone will not provide a complete picture of thyroid activity.

Remember, T4 merely measures the quantity of thyroid hormone *in the stored state*. It does not provide information as to whether that stored form is being accurately converted to the active form (T3). It does not provide information as to whether antibodies are attacking the thyroid hormone. And, it does not provide information as to whether sufficient thyroid stimulating hormone (thyroid's master hormone) is being produced.

To provide the clearest picture of thyroid function, experts recommend these tests:
    total T4 (tT4)
    free T4 by equilibrium dialysis (fT4ed: a very accurate method)
    total T3 (tT3)
    free T3
    T4 autoantibodies
    T3 autoantibodies

In addition, thyroglobulin autoantibodies (TgAA) and canine thyroid stimulating hormone (cTSH) tests may be recommended. The TSH test consists of drawing a baseline blood sample, after which, TSH (or synthetic formula) is administered by injection. Six hours later, a second blood sample is collected. The post-injection levels of thyroid hormone should be significantly higher. If they are not, thyroid gland dysfunction is indicated.

Abnormally high levels of TSH indicate that the body is trying to stimulate thyroid function. Active **autoimmune thyroid disease** typically presents elevated levels of TSH, low levels of free T4, and positive antibody tests. After the thyroid gland has been destroyed, antibody levels may drop.

AEDs, Cortisol, and Thyroid Tests

Cortisol and AED therapy can alter the results of some thyroid tests. Specifically, they can **suppress** the levels of the protein bound portion of Total T4 (tT4). This occurs even though the thyroid gland is working correctly. The *free* portion is believed to more accurately reflect true function of the gland but excess cortisol can lower this value, too.

In other cases, the opposite reaction occurs. Excess cortisol interferes with thyroid gland function *without* influencing test results. When tested, the results may indicate normal levels of thyroid hormone but they do not reveal that thyroid hormone has been **rendered inactive** by cortisol and adrenal estrogen.

It can be difficult to discern if hypothyroidism is a preexisting or coexisting condition, or if the symptoms are a result of AED therapy. Veterinary internists have developed the following protocol to address this situation.

> Each dog should be considered on an individual basis. If a dog is exhibiting signs of hypothyroidism, a six-week course of thyroid supplement should be administered. If, after six weeks, the clinical symptoms have diminished, it is likely that the dog was hypothyroid. If symptoms do not diminish, the treatment may be discontinued.

There is one other point to consider. If a dog has passed from excessive adrenal function to **adrenal exhaustion**, further complications present themselves. When a dog is treated with thyroid replacement hormone, the rate of metabolism rises. This increase can emphasize the adrenal insufficiency. Signs of lethargy and weakness may remain, leading to the false assumption that thyroid treatment was in error. In human healthcare, these patients are treated with both thyroid and adrenal replacement hormones. Thyroid levels should be rechecked about six weeks after therapy has started.

Hypothyroid Treatment

If your veterinarian diagnoses hypothyroidism, he will prescribe thyroid hormone supplements (pills) to be given once or twice each day. Most dogs require the latter, as thyroid supplements typically last 12 to 14 hours in dogs. Thyroid replacement hormone can have any number of trade names: Soloxine, Synthroid, or Eltroxin (in Canada). Studies indicate that human thyroid patients *do* react differently to individual brands and sometimes react better to name brands than to generic brands.

Thyroid replacement is typically considered a life-long therapy, although some dogs do seem to return to more normal thyroid function when chronic irritants (and cortisol levels) are reduced. As with most other endocrine disorders, hypothyroidism is a condition that is *treated*, not cured.

In Europe, human thyroid patients have access to **natural thyroid preparations** and **glandulars**: Dried, biological sources of the thyroid gland. Thyroid glandulars are less potent than prescription hormone replacement. They are sometimes available in dietary supplements (see Suppliers section) or through some holistic veterinarians.

Little scientific data exists on the efficacy of glandular extracts but it is interesting to note that studies done at the beginning of the 20th century indicated that human diabetics benefited from the oral ingestion of animal pancreas extracts. Eventually this work led scientists to the discovery and widespread use of injectable insulin, today's accepted treatment of Type 1 diabetes.

Thyroid hormone increases the activity rate of ATP production (metabolism), and increases the activity of sodium-potassium pump. This increase in metabolic activity seems to help some dogs return to more normal brain function. The owners of these dogs report a drop in seizure activity once hormone treatment has begun.

Dog owners often wonder about treating hypothyroidism through **dietary measures**. This is another situation in which a full thyroid panel provides valuable information. If the hypothyroidism is related to excess cortisol production, then certainly, feeding a more digestible, biologically appropriate diet is of value. This includes a diet with few grains or chemicals and one that contains at a minimum, some fresh food. In humans, grain intolerance has been linked to autoimmune thyroid disease. Eliminating grains cannot reverse the process but it may prevent additional autoimmune conditions from developing.

However, if the tests indicate that the hypothyroidism is *autoimmune* in nature, some dietary measures are less relevant. For example, some owners add kelp (iodine) to the diet, under the impression that it will aid hormone production. Supplementing iodine will be of little help, however, to the autoimmune patient, since the cells that once converted iodine into thyroid hormone have been destroyed.

Some experts recommend avoiding foods that produce goitrogens, substances that impair thyroid production. You may hear people cautioning against foods such as brussel sprouts, cauliflower, broccoli, spinach, and mustard greens. Avoiding cruciferous vegetables is less relevant to autoimmune thyroid patients since these vegetables are believed to interfere with thyroid *production*. If there are no thyroid cells, there is no production with which to interfere. However, some veterinarians still recommend this course of action since residual thyroid tissue may remain.

Ophthalmic Issues

It is interesting to note that a number of systemic diseases have an impact on ocular health. The eyes are delicate neural structures that succumb to the powerful effects of both the immune system and cortisol production.

It is extremely important to consult a veterinarian who specializes in ophthalmology at the onset of eye problems. Board-certified veterinary ophthalmologists are specifically trained to diagnosis and treat ophthalmic disease. They receive a minimum of four years of specialty education. This greatly differs from the few weeks of ophthalmic study that is provided in general veterinary training.

To discuss ophthalmic disease, a brief review of ocular anatomy will be helpful:

choroid — comprised mainly of blood vessels, one of the deep structural layers lining the back of the canine eye

ciliary body — the ocular structure that produces aqueous humor (the fluid in the eye); it is located just behind the iris

cornea — the transparent structure at the very front of the eye, which allows light to pass further into the globe

iris — the structure that acts as an aperture, constricting and dilating in size in response to the amount of light present

retina — the inner-most structural layer of nerve cells (rods and cones) that lines the back of the eye and sends visual information to the brain

tapetum — another of the structural layers lining the back of the canine eye that reflects and amplifies light

uvea (or uveal tract) — is made up of the iris, ciliary body, and choroid

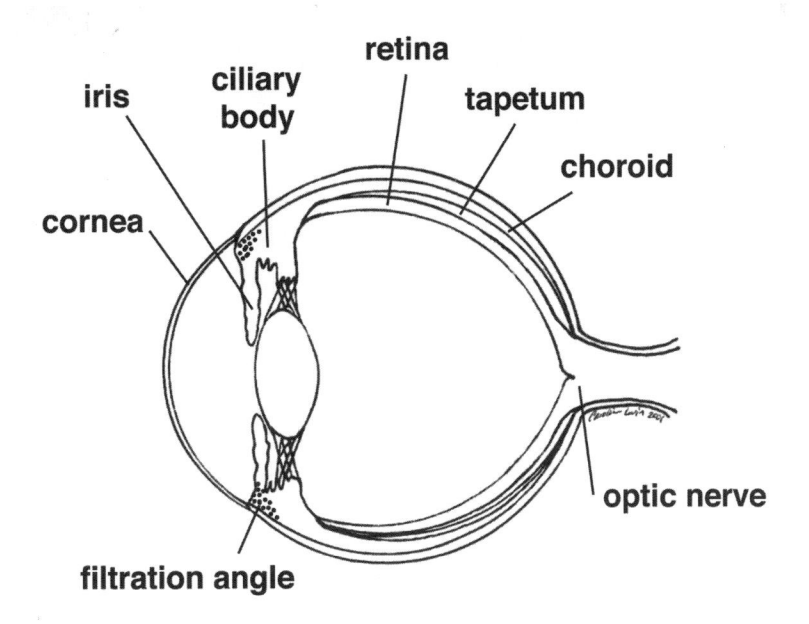

Eye diagram with labels: iris, ciliary body, retina, tapetum, choroid, cornea, optic nerve, filtration angle

Blindness Due to Transient Ischemia

Seizures that occur in the occipital lobe of the brain have long been associated with transient, bilateral blindness. You may hear this referred to as cortical blindness. It is unclear as to whether the blindness results from hypoxia of the cerebral brain cells or if the neuronal discharge disrupts visual recognition in some other way. Human epileptics report the presence of both blackouts and whiteouts following a seizure. Temporary blindness may last a few hours or days. (For additional resources, see page 192.)

Blindness Due to Sudden Acquired Retinal Degeneration Syndrome (SARD)

SARD involves an abrupt loss of vision and the deterioration of retinal cells in both eyes. Unlike cortical blindness, this deterioration is unrelated to seizure activity. As the name implies, the onset of blindness is *quite* sudden. Owners report that their dogs seem to go blind overnight.

SARD typically affects middle-aged animals often in the range of eight to ten years. It is frequently accompanied by other signs of excess cortisol production and usually results in complete and total blindness. It is not a physically painful condition.

This author submits that SARD is part of the "threefold effect" caused by commercial pet food. (See page 67.) As with dry eye syndrome and autoimmune thyroiditis, SARD *may* be an immune-mediated condition. But more likely, SARD is related to high levels of cortisol combined with inadequate nutrition. Specifically, this would include the inability of some dogs to metabolize fat and fat-soluble vitamins, such as A and E. MSG, the flavor enhancer present in many pet foods, damages the retinal cells of mice.

In humans, a gene called the p53 gene has been identified for its role in destroying damaged or mutated cells in the body. It does this by initiating a "self-destruct" message (or **apoptosis**) inside the damaged cell. This process normally prevents the growth of cancer.

Cellular damage occurs for a variety of reasons, including chemical damage, radiation exposure, and inadequate nutrition. When the body detects such damage to a cell, cortisol crosses the cell membrane and initiates the programmed, self-destruct message. If this process is similar in the canine body, then high levels of cortisol may be entering cells of the retina, damaged by inadequate nutrition, and programming them to self destruct.

There are recommended treatments for optic nerve inflammation and for brain cancer. At this time, there is no cure for SARD. A training program for blind dogs is the best form of treatment for dogs diagnosed with this condition. (See page 192.)

Dry Eye Syndrome (keratoconjunctivitis sicca or KCS)

As the name implies, dry eye syndrome results in reduced tear production, dryness, itchiness, and corneal ulcers. Another common sign of KCS is what owners term "goopy eyes," or the presence of green or light brown-colored mucous discharge. KCS is frequently misdiagnosed as an eye infection but antibiotic treatment does not resolve the problem.

KCS is yet another condition considered to have an immune-mediated basis. Antibodies that have been previously programmed to attack a foreign amino acid chain recognize and attack that same chain elsewhere in the body. In the case of KCS, the body attacks the tear-producing tissues of the eye.

KCS is commonly treated with cyclosporin drops. Cyclosporin is a medication thought to reduce the immune-mediated reaction. Other medications your veterinarian may prescribe are Optimmune drops or ointment (a milder form of cyclosporin), KCS drops, antibiotics, mucomyst (an ingredient that breaks up mucous), and a lubricant. Additional medications may include oral pilocarpine (which stimulates tear production), Natural Tears, or Lacrilube (lubricating drops and ointments that are available without a prescription).

Uveitis

Uveitis is the inflammation of the iris, ciliary body, or choroid. It can be caused by several factors, including an autoimmune reaction. Inflammation can occur in reaction to advanced cataracts or to other systemic inflammations (autoimmune disease) and infections.

Signs of uveitis include redness of the "whites of the eyes" (the conjunctiva), watery eyes, squinting, blinking, low intra-ocular pressure, and rubbing of the face on paws or the carpet. Pain can be expressed as depression or loss of appetite. Treatment usually requires steroid treatment, either with oral medication or eyedrops.

Glaucoma

Glaucoma is a condition of fluid build-up and abnormally high pressures within the eye. This usually occurs when the filtration angle (drainage field) no longer functions effectively. Left untreated, glaucoma can result in permanent, irreversible blindness, and pain. The early stages of glaucoma can include redness, cloudiness, bulging, a dilated pupil, and loss of vision. The dog may squint or rub his eye in an attempt to relieve pain.

The most common cause of glaucoma in dogs results from anatomical defects. In these cases, tissue blocks the filtration angle. As the dog ages, the tissue thickens, permitting less and less aqueous humor to escape. This type is called "primary" glaucoma. Injury or inflammation (such as uveitis) can also cause a blockage.

Treatment may initially include eye drops to reduce the pressure and detect whether or not the eye has any remaining vision. Unlike glaucoma in humans, eye drops and medications are usually not effective in the long-term treatment of *primary* glaucoma in dogs. Consequently, the veterinary ophthalmologist may recommend one of a variety of surgical procedures for your dog.

Note: Some epileptic dogs experience cluster seizures when methazolamide, a glaucoma medication, is prescribed in conjunction with phenobarbital. Methazolamide alters the rate at which other drugs are excreted.

Psychological Stress

Since psychological stress also releases cortisol, reducing this element may constitute another effective strategy for managing epilepsy.

Making a Safe Spot

Wolves and dogs are den animals. They retreat to small, protected places for safety, sleep, and rearing their young. Dens offer dogs a safe haven when they are tired or stressed. When dogs feel *un*safe, they stay trapped in the alarm phase of the stress adaptation response. They secrete more cortisol.

Create a safe spot for your epileptic. This may be an area separate from his nighttime sleeping spot. An ideal retreat for your dog would be a dog bed, dog-crate, or exercise pen (ex-pen). Place the bed or crate in an area where the family/pack spends most of its time, but avoid high-traffic paths. In this way, the dog can safely retreat from activity and not be isolated from social contact.

Some owners bristle at the idea of crating or "caging" a dog, but it is important to consider the issue from the dog's point of view. Many dogs are *more* comfortable when nestled into a small, sheltered space. It increases their sense of security and reduces their protective instinct.

If crating is a new experience for your dog, introduce him to the crate by throwing treats inside and letting him walk in and out. Try feeding him his dinner inside the crate. (Leave the door open, initially.) Do not forcibly push the dog inside the crate.

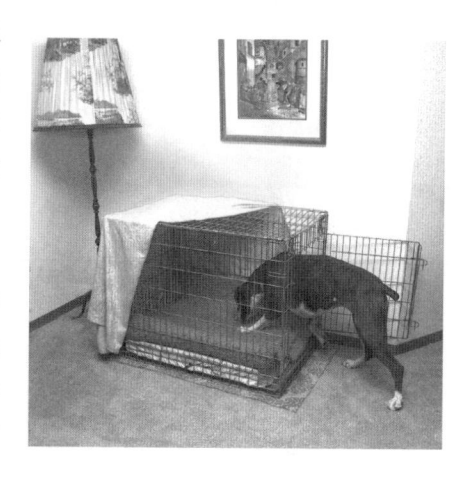

Crates are also an excellent solution for feeding raw chew bones as the smaller space reduces clean up. The same applies to incontinence. If you leave your dog for the length of a complete workday, ask a trusted friend, neighbor, or dog-sitting service to give the dog a potty break. Many adult dogs are content to sleep for an entire day, but younger dogs do best with a chance to stretch their legs.

It is possible that other dogs in your household will seek out the epileptic's safe spot. In this case, beds may be in order for everyone! The key is to enforce each dog's right to a place he can always call his own. This may mean verbally correcting other dogs or physically removing them. Households with multiple dogs have been quite successful in maintaining designated resting spots. In some households, this type of territorialism may not be a problem at all.

Pack Issues

The normal canine social structure is the pack. Many people do not realize the all-encompassing importance pack life has for a dog. The organization of the pack governs most canine behaviors, communications, and welfare.

Wolves have existed in packs for thousands of years. Typically there is a male leader called an alpha (meaning first) dog. There is also an alpha female. The remainder of the pack is structured in a descending hierarchy — a beta male and female, a gamma male and female, and so on.

Wolf packs are obviously made up of wolves. Domesticated dogs may have several different species in their packs. These may include other dogs, humans, and, in some instances, cats or farm animals. Domesticated packs typically have a leader amongst the dogs, as well as a human leader positioned over the entire pack. It is best if all humans, including children, have more dominant roles in the pack.

In human society, we like to think of all men as being "created equal." In the dog pack, this is not so. We need to accept this, difficult as it may be. The pack is structured in such a way as to promote cooperation and ensure the survival of its members. If all dogs or wolves were equals, there would be no distinct leader to protect the pack from danger. A dog's position in the pack is decided by several factors, such as age, the dog's basic personality, and how the other pack members react to a dog.

Dogs that rank higher in the pack (more dominant) are entitled to more privileges. They get the best sleeping places and expect other pack members to move out of their way. They walk through doorways, first. Dominant dogs defend their food and may steal the food or toys of other dogs. Other displays of dominance include placing a paw or chin across another dog's back, standing over or mounting another dog, growling, and marking territory with urine.

Submissive dogs range from beta (a happy-go-lucky individual that might take on a leadership role if circumstances dictated) to omega, a sometimes fearful, anxious dog. Submissive dogs yield to more dominant pack members. They roll over on their back, relinquish toys, food, and their sleeping places.

Submission is not synonymous with cowardice or punishment. In the dog's culture, it is a form of cooperation. It is important for us to realize that dogs are content with this arrangement. They typically don't mind being in any particular pack position, they simply wish to know *where* they rank. In fact, dogs are *most comfortable* when they know their position and that position maintains consistency.

Humans create a sense of safety and well being for their dogs when they communicate in consistent ways. Unfortunately, many people do not effectively communicate their leadership to their dogs. These owners may give verbal commands but may not enforce them. They may back down if their dog growls at them. They may routinely put the dog's wishes before their own.

As humans, we usually want others to like us. We may feel uncomfortable enforcing rules to our beloved pets. Dogs don't view things this way. Their comfort and security comes from an orderly and structured social setting. We do our dogs a kindness when we behave as strong leaders.

Inconsistent behaviors (those that are not consistent with the alpha position) from the human are confusing to the dog. If a dog concludes that there is no real pack-leader, his instinct will be to rise to that position himself. This instinct would insure the continued survival of the wild pack. It also represents the core of many behavioral problems we see in domesticated dogs, today. When a dog doesn't consider his human pack members to be higher ranking, the dog may challenge them in an attempt to take control himself.

Separation Anxiety

In the wild, there is safety in remaining close to other pack members, especially when out on the hunt. If a single wolf is separated from the pack, he becomes vulnerable to attack by other animals. This may explain a little bit about the separation anxiety experienced by so many domesticated dogs when their owners leave the house without them.

It is alarming for some dogs to be without the other members of their pack. When it is necessary to leave your dog, distracting him with a new toy or chew bone can help allay his fears. Leave a radio or television turned on. Having other companions at home, canine or feline, may help some dogs.

Various training programs encourage owners to leave and return at varying time intervals to increase the dog's self-confidence. Leave for a minute or two and then return. If his behavior was good, reward him. (It may be necessary to set up a video camera or enlist the help of a hidden friend to discern the dog's behavior. In other cases, the damage is apparent.) Gradually lengthen the time you are gone. Do not make a big scene when you leave. Behave calmly and do not fuss over the dog.

Crating is another method of dealing with separation anxiety. As previously described, dogs are den animals that seek small, sheltered spaces for safety. When dogs feel safe, they are typically less destructive. Initially, some dogs may object to the crate. This, too, is related to separation anxiety. Be patient and consistent.

Even with the best training programs, it can be difficult to manage separation anxiety. Anxiety in modern dogs may be a combination of both mental and physical elements including metabolism, stress hormones, and neurochemicals. Reconsider switching the dog to a natural diet if you have not already done so.

Changes in Pack Dynamics

Mental stress also stems from changes in pack dynamics, that is, the addition of a new member or when one matures into adulthood. Some behaviorists recommend that you allow dogs to determine pack order by themselves. Other experts believe that, as the *true* pack leader, it is best for the owner to forbid any type of dog fighting or aggression.

The stress of a new dog may trigger seizures, so maintaining the older dog's mental peace can be beneficial. If the epileptic has always been the dominant dog, it may be worthwhile to help him retain his position. It is your job to enforce good manners in your pack. If your dogs believe you are the true pack leader, they will respond to your household rules.

In the wild, dominant wolves eat first from the prey they have killed. You can promote a dog's dominant position by feeding him dinner prior to the other dogs. For serious cases, you can feed him a special treat or biscuit in front of, but not including, the other dogs.

Since dominant dogs typically pass through doorways before subordinate dogs, encourage the epileptic dog through the door first. This may require physically restraining the other dog or dogs while verbally encouraging the epileptic. If this proves too difficult, you might prefer allowing the top dog outdoors separately from the others.

Make sure the alpha dog has a special, more privileged bed or sleeping place. Since people all live differently with their dogs, "special" can take on different meanings.

Regardless of where or how your dogs sleep at night, the closer the sleeping spot is to *you*, the more privileged a position it is. If your dogs sleep outside, an indoor sleeping spot would be a privileged position over the other dogs. If the dogs sleep indoors, sleeping in the bedroom, or on the bed would be the privilege.

Traveling

If you are traveling without your dog, try to arrange for him to stay in his own environment with the help of friends, family members, or the services of a professional house sitter. This may be the least stressful option for your dog. Commercial kennels are fraught with stress as unfamiliar dogs are kept in close quarters. Minimizing stress may minimize seizure activity. On the other hand, if your dog should have a seizure while you were away, a 24-hour veterinary clinic kennel would be the best place to attain immediate attention.

If you are traveling *with* your dog, avoid exposure to extremes of weather. Dehydration, heat, and exhaustion can increase seizure activity. Avoid transporting epileptics in airline cargo holds. It is stressful in a number of ways. If you are going to stay in a hotel with the dog, practice before you go. If a motel or hotel in your area accepts dogs, it may be possible for you to expose him to hotel lobbies, elevators, etc., before the actual trip.

Competitive Sports and the Epileptic

As previously discussed, moderate exercise can be an effective method of managing stress and reducing seizure activity. Dog trainers worldwide recognize the mental health benefits that dogs derive from "having a job." However, competitive canine sports are a slightly different matter. Obedience matches, hunting trials, and agility competitions can be highly stressful situations.

In these environments, dogs are often kept in close quarters. Some respond with aggressive behaviors. Loud noises are routine: Dogs bark, applause bursts out, and loudspeakers blare. Energy levels are high and owners themselves may transmit a sense of stress to their dogs.

If your dog seizes during or after a competition, a change in activities may be in order. Sometimes this means switching to a less stressful sport or training technique. Positive and motivational training methods are less stressful than older, more punitive types involving heavy collar and verbal corrections. Chronically high levels of cortisol are known to damage learning ability in humans. If your dog seems to be having difficulty understanding your commands, review the options for lowering cortisol production.

All that being said, a number of epileptic dogs have highly successful careers in competitive sports. They enjoy daily training, compete regularly, and earn titles. This is a testament to the quality of life an epileptic dog can lead.

Lorbach's Liza Do Lots AKC UDX, CKC UD, pictured at age 10, earned her advanced Utility Dog Excellent title a year and a half after her first seizure.

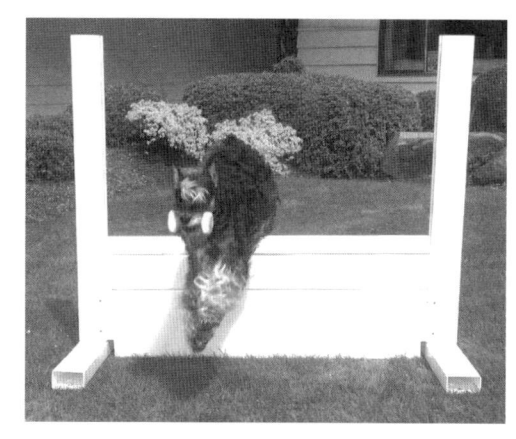

Photo courtesy of Joeanne Butler

Other Factors That Contribute to Canine Disease

In addition to a faulty, irritating diet and a genetic predisposition, several other factors are believed to contribute to immune system failure and endocrine disease. Environmental toxins and over-vaccination are two of these.

Heartworm Prevention

In certain parts of the world, the threat of heartworm infestation is very real. Warm climates provide the right environment for mosquito populations, the carriers of heartworm larvae. If you do not live in a high risk area, or wish to reduce the chemical insult to your dog, there are other methods of preventing serious injury or death from heartworms.

Transmission of heartworm is dependent upon the lifecycle of the mosquito. Studies indicate that daily, average temperatures must exceed 64 F (18 C) for approximately one month, in order to support the mosquito lifecycle. Another source suggests that temperatures must exceed 80 F (27 C) for at least two weeks. If temperatures fall below 57 F (14 C), the lifecycle is interrupted. Using these guidelines, it may not be necessary to treat for heartworms year round, in all locales.

Heartworm medications are *treatments* not preventatives. They slowly kill circulating larvae. They do not prevent the dog from contracting an infestation in the first place. With that in mind, some dog owners begin treatment one month after temperatures reach 64 F and continue until one month after temperatures drop below 57 F.

Other owners don't use any medications and simply test twice yearly. However, **routine testing is *crucial*** to prevent infestation. Without these twice-yearly checks an infestation can become uncontrolled and life-threatening. If the test results are positive, your veterinarian will likely take an x-ray to determine the level of infestation. Mild infestations caught early are often treated with the same medications used on a monthly or daily basis. These are sometimes termed "slow kill" medications. Advanced infestations are much more serious, requiring treatment in the veterinary hospital. This may include "fast kill" medications and IV fluids.

If you and your veterinarian feel year round preventives are mandatory, some products may be more suitable than others for epileptics. Dr. R. Clemmons believes products such as Filarbits and Interceptor are safer for epileptic dogs. Additionally, some owners report lower seizure activity on plain tablet medications versus chewable forms. Chewable tablets have additional **flavorings** that some suspect as the cause of this problem.

Flea Control

There are many options for more wholesome flea control. Vacuum one to three times, weekly. Wash the dog's bedding frequently. Use a flea comb regularly, dipping the comb into a bowl of soapy water to drown any fleas you find. Most soaps will kill fleas.

Bathe your dog regularly but avoid shampoos that contain pyrethrins. Although these are specifically designed to kill fleas they do so by *interfering with neurological function*. There are ever-increasing numbers of herbal repellants and natural shampoos available. (It may be best for epileptics to *avoid* those with the strong fragrances of essential oils.)

Control flea populations by keeping lawns short and leaves raked. Apply predatory nematodes (simple roundworms that devour insects) or diatomaceous earth (a calcium dust that acts as a natural insecticide) to lawns. These are available at many garden centers.

Cedar chips should be used with caution around epileptics. Cedar, like pine, contains phenols — chemicals known to disrupt endocrine function and lower the seizure threshold. Be alert for the presence of cedar chips in commercial kennels and pet beds. Be sure to evaluate your dog's physical condition if you introduce cedar chips to the environment. Certain sensitive individuals may exhibit increased seizures, and young puppies may exhibit allergic symptoms to cedar.

Certain dietary supplements may be helpful in discouraging fleas. These include B vitamin complex and small amounts of garlic. And don't forget the basic benefits of a more natural diet. Pests tend to infest animals that have diminished resistance. Dogs are compromised when fed difficult-to-digest commercial food. It weakens their immune system. Owners treat the resultant infestations with chemicals that likely *worsen* their immune system and neural function. Many owners report reduced flea problems after a switch to fresh food.

If you absolutely must use pesticide flea treatments on your dog, try to prolong the period between applications. It may be possible to apply a product only several times yearly rather than every thirty days. Make a note in your seizure journal when you apply flea treatments to your dog.

New Vaccine Protocols

More and more veterinarians are moving away from the practice of annual vaccines for the duration of a dog's life. There is a greater awareness of the potential harm vaccines may cause to immunologically compromised dogs. If your dog is an adult (over three to four years of age) and is epileptic, it may be beneficial to avoid any further vaccines not required by law. In serious cases, your veterinarian may even be able to write your dog a waiver, exempting him from rabies vaccines.

The most current vaccine recommendations vary depending on the source. However, some basic principles are shared. Following an initial series of puppy vaccines (typically a series of three), a booster may be given one year later and every *three years*, thereafter.

Most vaccines available on the market today are prepared as *combo* vaccines. In other words, four or five antigens (such as parvovirus, parainfluenza, distemper, etc.) are combined in a single injection. While this is convenient, it is also extremely demanding on the body to mount an immune response to each antigen at the same time.

Holistic veterinarians often recommend giving vaccines as "split components" or individual injections. Furthermore, individual puppy vaccines should be given at intervals separated by several weeks or months. This allows the immune system a reasonable recovery period.

Adult boosters of individual components can be separated by one-year intervals. In other words, the veterinarian may recommend that your adult dog receive a parvo booster one year, a distemper booster the next year, and a rabies booster the year after.

Additionally, consider that your dog may not be at risk for every single disease for which vaccines exist. As owners become more discriminating in their dog's healthcare some are steering away from having their dog receive every vaccine on the market. This is especially true if a particular disease is geographically related.

Lengthy discussion exists as to the pros and cons of using vaccines that contain "killed" organisms versus those that contain "modified live" organisms. While killed vaccines cause less strain on the dog's system, there exists some concern that they may not impart sufficient protection. Please discuss all of these concepts with your veterinarian.

Another way to minimize unnecessary vaccines is to request that your veterinarian "measures titers." This involves drawing a small amount of blood and having it tested for its reactivity to the antigens in question. Titers do not offer a complete picture of the dog's immune status, but they give the best information currently available. If titer levels return "good to excellent," it is likely unnecessary to revaccinate the individual against that disease.

Surgical Considerations

Preparation for a surgical procedure can play havoc with a dog's stress level. Most often, dog owners are instructed to withhold food from midnight on, before the day of surgery. Consequently, dogs that experience hypoglycemia may be at an increased risk of having seizures. Ask your veterinarian if you may administer a spoonful of ice cream and/or herbal remedy on the morning of the procedure. Try to reduce stress with massage.

Certain sedatives, tranquilizers, and anesthetics (particularly Acepromazine and Ketamine) can be problematic for epileptics. Remind the veterinary staff that your dog is epileptic prior to any treatment he receives.

Epilepsy and Breeding Practices

There are two primary reasons why dogs with idiopathic epilepsy should not be bred. The first reason is in the interest of the puppies. Clearly there appears to be a genetic tendency towards epilepsy in some breeds and some familial lines. Breeding epileptic dogs may result in an increased number of epileptics in the canine population.

The second reason involves the brood bitch. Estrogen levels rise during pregnancy and increased estrogen is linked with an increase in seizure activity. It is in the best interest of epileptic bitches to exclude them from a breeding program. Discuss with your veterinarian the benefits of spaying such animals.

Breeders are often interested in discerning which of their breeding stock contribute to cases of inherited epilepsy. This problem appears to involve multiple genes, so simple testing measures do not appear imminent. However, research is currently underway through the Canine Epilepsy Project. The goal of this collaborative study is to identify the genes responsible for epilepsy in dogs and promote wise breeding decisions. It is supported by grants from the AKC Canine Health Foundation, National Institutes of Health, individual breed clubs, and private donations.

Comfort Measures

There are a number of additional ways to comfort dogs. The following suggestions are aimed at dogs experiencing the effects of excess cortisol or the steroid-like affects of phenobarbital.

Heat Intolerance

Help your dog manage heat intolerance by offering him a cool place to rest. This can be a small plastic pool in the yard, frozen water bottles in his crate, or cooling pads in the house. Cooling pads are available commercially or can be homemade. Some contain polymer crystals that are soaked in water.

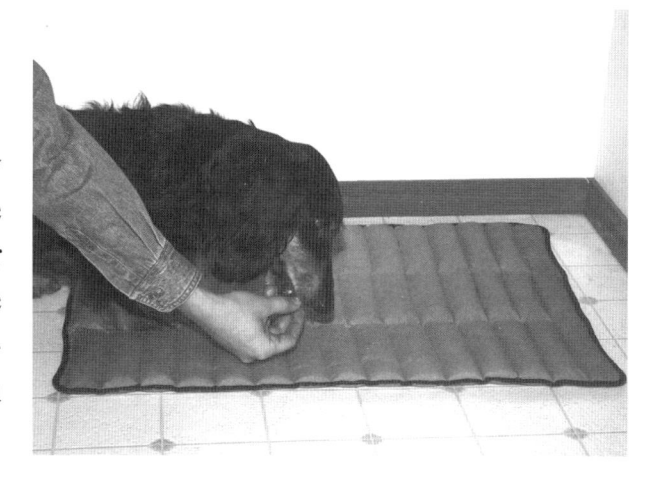

Some pads are *filled* with water or other coolants. (One owner placed dry, frozen soup beans inside a pillowcase.) This style may be more attractive to some dogs since the pads are cool but still dry to the touch. (See Supplier's section.) These pads may also be more attractive to owners since they can be placed on wall-to-wall carpeting without causing damage.

If you can sew, you can make your own cooling pad with heavy cotton fabric and polymer granules available at plant nurseries. These granules absorb enormous amounts of water.

Instructions:
Cut the fabric to the size pad appropriate for your dog. Sew around three sides. Sew parallel tubes about 1.5 inches wide. Place approximately one teaspoon of granules for each 12 inches of tube length. Then sew across the fourth side of the mat, closing off all the tubes. Soak the pad in cool water for about 30 minutes. Refrigerate the mat when it becomes too warm. Completely dry the mat if you need to remove or add more crystals.

Even though your dog will eventually appreciate the cooling pad, he may be reluctant to use it at first. Introduce your dog to the cooling pad with food treats. Do not force him onto the pad. Initially, feed him near the pad. Later, place treats on the pad. If he places a foot on it, reward him with praise and additional treats. As you repeat this experience, the dog will come to view the pad as a positive thing. He will become less apprehensive and eventually begin to use it.

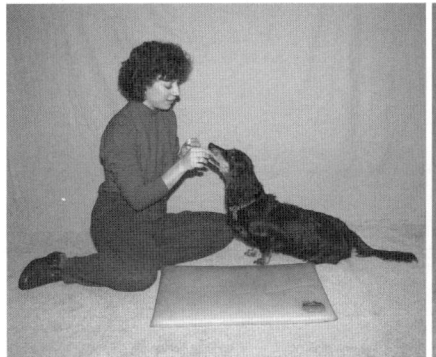

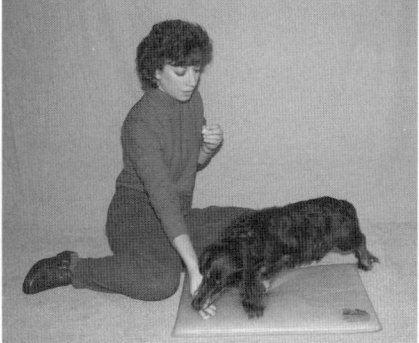

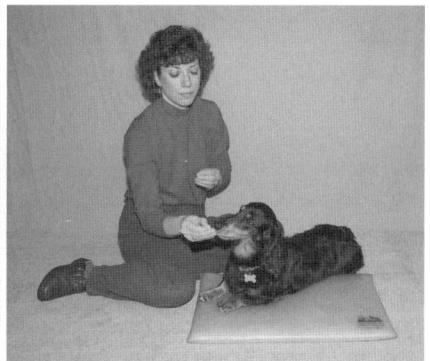

Muscle Weakness

Many owners implement the use of ramps and footstools for their dogs with muscle weakness. Footstools can be used to help a dog make the transition from floor to furniture, and vice versa. (The footstool pictured at right is actually a small wicker chest covered with a bath mat.) Ramps can also be used in such situations, as well as for access to automobiles and to negotiate partial flights of stairs.

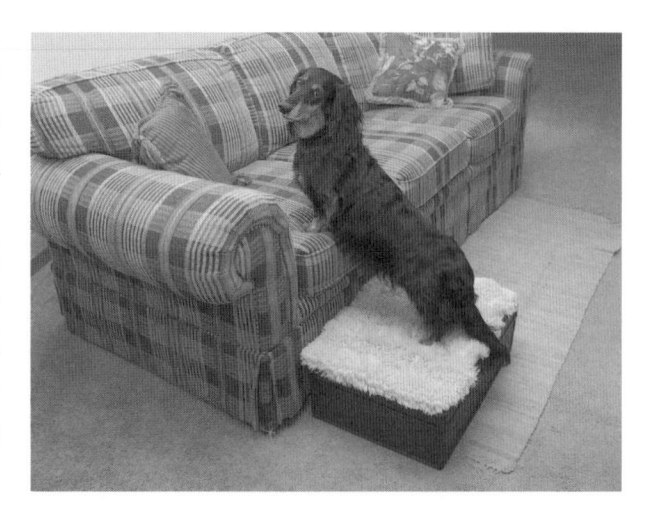

If you pursue such an option, enlist the skills of an experienced carpenter or builder (or see Suppliers list). It would be detrimental to the dog's self-confidence to have a ramp collapse or slip out from under him. Tack down outdoor carpeting or anti-skid tape such as that found on commercial building stairways. Consider building a wall or safety railing to keep the dog from inadvertently stepping off the side of the ramp. The longer the flight of stairs, the longer the ramp must be.

Introduce your dog to the ramp with a food treat held close to his nose. If he is reluctant to step onto the ramp, dab on bits of peanut butter or cream cheese up the ramp in a row. Offer him verbal encouragement to help him find each succeeding treat.

If you have wooden, tile, or linoleum flooring, purchase gripper socks, rubber mats, or carpet runners with rubber backing. The latter are available at home-improvement stores, carpet stores, and some hardware stores. They can be cut in half width-wise to accommodate small dogs and be more cost-effective.

Place an additional mat at the dog's food bowl. This will offer him extra security. You can also provide your dog with raised food and water bowls, which may contribute to steadiness on his feet.

Assist large, weak, or unsteady dogs down the stairs by slipping a towel under their belly to serve as a sling. You can use a canvas log-carrier (the type found at fireplace shops) as they often are constructed with handles. And, you can even purchase slings designed specifically for pets. (See Suppliers section.) These techniques can also help weak dogs manage slick floors at the veterinary clinic or grooming shop.

References

Barry, E., et al, "Ictal Blindness and Status Epilepticus Amauroticus," *Epilepsi*a, 26(6): 1985.

Berti, I., et al, "Usefulness of Screening Program for Celiac Disease in Autoimmune Thyroiditis," *Digestive Diseases and Sciences,* 45(2): February, 2000.

Carlson, D.G., and Giffin, J.M., *Dog Owner's Home Veterinary Handbook.* New York: Howell Book House, 1992.

Clemmons, R.M., "Seizure Disorders in Dogs and Cats," http://pawcare.com/rclemmons, January, 2002.

Colorado State University Veterinary Teaching Hospital, "Small Animal Vaccination Protocol," http://www.vth.colostate.edu/vth/savp2.html, February, 2002.

Dodds, W.J., "Autoimmune Thyroid Disease," *DogWorld,* 77(5): October, 1992.

Dudley, K., "Eliminate Fleas Without Poisons: Integrated Pest Management is a Nontoxic Way to Effectively Control Fleas," *Whole Dog Journal,* 5(3): March, 2002.

Johnstone, C., Knight, D.H., and Lok, J.B., "Epidemiology of Canine Heartworm Disease," http://cal.vet.upenn.edu/parasit/heartworm/hw_3.html, July, 1997.

Kantrowitz, L.B., "Serum Total Thyroxin, Total Triiodothyronine, Free Thyroxin and Thyroxin and Thyrotropin Concentrations in Epileptic Dogs Treated with Anticonvulsants," *Journal of the American Veterinary Medical Association,* 214(12): June, 1999.

Levin, C.D., *Dogs, Diet, and Disease: An Owner's Guide to Diabetes Mellitus, Pancreatitis, Cushing's Disease, and More.* Oregon City: Lantern Publications, 2001.

Natori, Y., et al, "Changes of Thyroid Hormone Levels During ACTH Therapy in Epileptic Children," *Rinsho Byori,* (article originally in Japanese) July, 1994.

Northwest Coalition for Alternatives to Pesticides (NCAP) staff, "Managing Fleas Without Poisons," *Journal of Pesticide Reform,* 17(3): Fall, 1997.

Raber, J., "Detrimental Effects of Chronic Hypothalamic-Pituitary-Adrenal Axis Activation," *Molecular Neurobiology,* August, 1998.

Richard, A., and Reiter, J., *Epilepsy: A New Approach.* New York: Prentice Hall, 1990.

Shames, R., and Shames K.H., *Thyroid Power: Ten Steps to Total Health.* New York: Harper Resource, 2001.

Wolfsheimer, K., "Thyroid Testing in Dogs: A Reference for Dog Breeders and Owners," an article from the Louisiana State University School of Veterinary Medicine http://www.golden-retriever.com/thyr-lsu.html, November, 2001.

Chapter 12

Closing Thoughts

Emotional Support

Caring for dogs with chronic medical conditions is a labor of love. It can be emotionally exhausting. Not all of your friends, family, and co-workers will understand your commitment. Try to surround yourself with those who do.

Try to enjoy small pleasures with your dog and do not forget to take some time off for yourself and your own mental health. Enlist the help of others if you need a break from the role of caregiver. Burnout is a common side effect of providing long-term care.

A Word About Dog Training

Canine behaviors are best taught or modified by positive means, not punishment. If you are having difficulty dealing with your dog, first identify the problem behavior. Then, using food treats, show the dog what you want him to do differently. Food and toys are powerful rewards for dogs.

If your dog views a situation as unpleasant or frightening, offer him food treats lavishly during that time. The dog will come to view the event as a rewarding experience. Be generous with your rewards. It's a good way to go through life.

The Future

Every pet owner faces the day when his dog will be lost to illness, age, or injury. It is a painful time for any animal lover. There are many good books devoted to the subject of pet loss; therefore, this topic will not be discussed at length here. However, the following story is offered in the hope that it provides the reader some small measure of comfort when that day arrives.

The Rainbow Bridge

There is a bridge connecting Heaven and Earth. It is called the Rainbow Bridge because of its many colors. Just this side of the Rainbow Bridge, there is a land of meadows, hills, and valleys with lush green grass.

When a beloved pet dies, the pet goes to this place. There is always food and water and warm spring weather. The old and frail animals are young again. Those who are maimed are made whole again. They play all day with each other.

There is only one thing missing. They are not with their special person who loved them on Earth. So, each day they run and play until the day comes when one suddenly stops playing and looks up. The nose twitches. The ears are up. The eyes are staring. And this one suddenly runs from the group!

You have been seen and when you and your special friend meet, you take him or her in your arms and embrace. Your face is kissed again and again and again, and you look once more into the eyes of your trusting pet. Then you cross the Rainbow Bridge together, never again to be separated.

— Author Unknown

Some dog owners turn to new methods of animal husbandry after losing a pet to chronic illness. They embark on a more natural approach to dog feeding and healthcare. If you, too, are of this philosophy, seek out like-minded dog breeders. They can provide you with a puppy that has never been fed commercial food. This is important, since some of the most crucial damage appears to occur early in life. If you prefer mixed breeds, it is sometimes possible to adopt young puppies from animal shelters.

Whether your canine companions are puppies or adults, may your lives together be long. The human-canine bond is precious. None of us should lose a dog prematurely and none of our pets should needlessly suffer.

A hidden connection is stronger than an obvious one.
— Heraclitus c. 500 BC

Suppliers and Resources

Internet discussion groups:

http://www.canine-epilepsy.com
Canine epilepsy resource center: articles, links, etc. List-serve (mailing list) for owners of epileptic dogs.

http://www.canine-epilepsy-guardian-angels.com
Epilepsy resource pages, articles, links, etc. One-on-one email support from experienced epileptic-dog owners. Mailing list by invitation.

http://groups.yahoo.com/group/k9epilepsy/

Suppliers:

American Eagle Food Machinery, Inc.
3557 South Halsted Street
Chicago, IL 60609-1606
Phone: (773) 376-0800
Toll free phone numbers:
    Order Hotline: (800) 836-5756, Customer Service: (888) 390-0800
Web site: http://www.americaneaglemachine.com

Retailers of commercial-grade stainless steel meat/bone grinders

---

American Nutrition
5092 Buttercup Drive
Castle Rock, CO 80104
Toll Free (800) 454-3724
International (303) 814-9879
Web site: http://www.americannutrition.com/Natures_Purest/natures_purest.htm

Distributors of Purest Brand Phosphatidyl Serine, which is reportedly 99% pure. Select "Purest Products" on their webpage.

Aunt Jeni's Home Made Dog Food
PO Box 124
Temple Hills, MD 20757
Toll free: (877) 254-6123
Web site: http://www.auntjeni.com

In Canada:
Pets4Life
RR #4
Owen Sound, ONT N4K 5N6
Phone: (519) 372-1818

Makers and distributors of *Home Made 4 Life* brand dog food, a premixed, frozen Bones And Raw Food diet.

Azmira Holistic Animal Care & Nutritional Products
2100 North Wilmot Road, Suite 109
Tucson, AZ 85712
Phone: (520) 886-8548
Toll free: (800) 497-5665
Web site: http://www.azmira.com

Holistic digestive aids: vitamin/mineral supplements, digestive enzymes, herbal formulas such as: Panc'rse & Glucobalance drops, Herbal Calm, Calm & Relax, Stress & A'drenal Plex extract, Immuno Stim'r drops, and kidney/urinary tract formulas, canned and kibbled dog and cat food with human-grade meat.

B-Naturals
Natural and Holistic Supplements for Dogs and Cats
PO Box 217
Rockford, MN 55373
Phone: (763) 477-7001
Toll free (United States): (866) 368-2728
Web site: http://www.b-naturals.com

Braggs Organic Apple Cider Vinegar, PurePet Oatmeal Shampoo, SAMe, Bertes Immune Blend Vitamins. Herbs and herbal formulas: Skin and Liver Plex, Kidni-Biotic, Kidni-Care, Cranberry Extract, Immune System Formula, HAC Immuno Stim'r, HAC Yeast and Fungal, HAC Blood & Lymph, HAC Stress & Adrenal, and Milk Thistle. Digestive enzymes (Berte's Di-Acid Dim) and Berte's Ultra Probiotic Powder. Essential fatty acids such as Flax, Borage and Salmon Oil Caps.

Brandt P.P. Pants
715 Brandywine Drive
Lodi, CA 95240
Phone: (209) 368-6810
Web site: http://www.lodinet.com/pppants

Diapers for male dogs.

C & D Pet Products
405 East D Street
Petaluma, CA 94952
Phone: (707) 763-1654
Toll free: (888) 554-7387
Web site: http://www.cdpets.com

Carpeted pet steps, single or double, to help pets access furniture.

Choose to Heel
10409 Canyon Road E.
Suite 263
Puyallup, WA 98373
http://www.choosetoheel.com

Highly motivational, low-stress, competitive dog training theory. Classes, seminars, books and videos presented by Dawn Jecs, nationally recognized obedience/agility instructor, competitor, and lecturer.

Commercial Matting/Consolidated Plastics Company, Inc.
8181 Darrow Road
Twinsburg, OH 44087
Toll free: (800) 362-1000

Mats and carpet runners with rubber backing.

Doctors Foster & Smith Inc.
2253 Air Park Road
Rhinelander, WI 54501-0100
Toll free: (800) 826-7206
Web site: http://www.drsfostersmith.com

Housebreaking pads, folding ramps for accessing trucks and RVs, dental care kits, Pet Pectate diarrhea control, urinary acidifier, pet bloomers and fancy pants (diapers for females), raised water and food bowls, and Rescue Remedy.

Four Flags Over Aspen, Inc.
P.O. Box 190
St. Clair, MN 56080
Toll free: (800) 222-9263
Web site: http://www.fourflags.com/FFOA-3.html#fleece

Makers of the Soft Quick Lift, a fleece-lined body sling to carry animals.

Holistic Pet Center
The Health Food Store for Pets
PO Box 1166 or 15599 SE 82nd Drive
Clackamas, OR 97015
Phone: (503) 656-5342
Web site: http://www.holisticpetcenter.com

Makers and distributors of Vetline "Calm" herbal formula and Vetline Vitamins, which include, among other things, amino acids and glandular extracts. (Not for use with raw meaty bone diets however, as this would result in excess calcium.)

---

iHerb Inc.
1435 S. Shamrock Avenue
Monrovia, CA 91016
Phone: (626) 358-5678
Toll Free (8:00 am to 6:00 pm PST): (888) 792-0028
Website: http://www.iherb.com

Distributors of Jarrow brand Phosphatidyl Serine. Search webpage with: "PS."

I.Q. Industries Inc.
737 Park Avenue
New York, NY 10021
Toll free: (877) 364-5438
Web site: http://www.dogramp.com

Heavy-duty, one-piece dog ramps with carpeting.

Maverick Marketing Ventures, Inc.
12550 Wolff Street
Broomfield, CO 80020
Phone: (303) 410-9020
Toll free (United States): (888) 244-5569
Web site: http://www.soothsoft.com

Canine Cooler Brand Thermoregulation Pet Bet — available in a variety of sizes and filled with water but due to their design, do not require refrigeration to keep pets cool.

Natural Pets
PO Box 1461
Point Roberts, WA 98281-1461
Phone: (604) 591-6168
Web site: http://www.naturalpets.net
Contact Natural Pets for their Canadian mailing address.

Distributors of a range of natural nutritional supplements and herbal formulas.

Pinnacle Pet Supply
7251 PR 241 Mprtj
Cartier, MB R4K 1B4 Canada
Toll free (Canada): (877) 968-7738
Toll free (United States): (877) 668-7770
Web site: http://www.escape.ca/~pps/kooler.html

Kanine Kooler Pad — a 12" x 18" vinyl bag that is filled with water. It only weighs about 5 lbs., but it must be refrigerated to remain cool.

Purely Pets
4240 Daniels Street
Chester, VA 23831
Phone: (804) 748-7626
Web site: http://www.purelypets.com

Makers of Epi Plus — a natural herb and vitamin supplement for epileptic dogs.

SleePee-Time Beds
2730 Willow Oak Circle
Charlottesville, VA 22901
Phone: (804) 296-1683
Toll free: (888) 824-7705
Web site: http://www.sleepeetime.com

Pet bed designed for incontinent animals.

Standard Process Whole Food Supplements
Standard Process Inc.
1200 West Royal Lee Drive
PO Box 904
Palmyra, WI 53156-0904
Phone: (262) 495-2122
Toll free: (800) 848-5061 (USA)
Web site: http://www.standardprocess.com/index.asp

Suppliers of veterinary supplements including immune system support and glandular extracts. Ask your veterinarian for assistance.

Glossary

absence seizure — a momentary loss of consciousness

Acidophilus — beneficial bacteria available as a dietary supplement

ACTH stimulation test — adrenocorticotrophic hormone stimulation test that indicates the presence of Cushing's Disease

adipose — fatty body tissue

adrenal glands — two small endocrine glands located near the kidneys that secrete cortisol and adrenaline, as well as several other important hormones

adrenocorticotrophic hormone (ACTH) — produced by the pituitary gland and responsible for cortisol secretion via the adrenal glands

AEDs — antiepileptic drugs such as phenobarbital or potassium bromide

ALKP — alkaline phosphatase, a liver enzyme

ALT — alanine aminotransferase, a liver enzyme

amino acids — the building blocks of protein

amylase — a pancreatic enzyme responsible for digesting carbohydrates

apoptosis — programmed cell death

aspartate — an excitatory neurotransmitter and amino acid derived from aspartic acid

ataxia — loss of muscle co-ordination

atrophy — withering of tissues and organs

aura — unusual sensations that warn of an impending seizure

autoimmune disease (or immune-mediated condition) — a condition in which the immune system destroys the body's own cells and tissues

BID — twice daily

bilateral — both sides

bile — a salty, yellowish fluid produced by the liver, stored in the gall bladder, necessary for the digestion of dietary lipids

bilirubin — a bile pigment derived from the breakdown of hemoglobin

bio-availability — a measure of how well nutrients are used by the body

catabolism — the effect cortisol has in breaking down muscle tissue to supply the body with glucose and amino acids

celiac disease — an intolerance to wheat gluten/protein that may accompany autoimmune disease and epilepsy

channels — molecular "gates" (proteins) within cell membranes that control the flow of ions in and out of a cell

clonic seizures — seizures that cause repeated jerking movements

cluster seizure — seizures occurring close together, over a period of several days or hours

complex partial seizures — seizures involving only one part of the brain but which results in a loss or change of consciousness

cortisol — a natural steroid/hormone produced by the adrenal glands that is primarily responsible for ensuring the presence of glucose in the bloodstream

CT (computerized tomography) — a brain scan that reveals brain structure

Cushing's disease — the pituitary-dependent form of hyperadrenocorticism (HAC) first identified by Dr. Harvey Cushing

EEG (electroencephalogram) — a clinic test that records brain waves

electrolytes — substances such as sodium, potassium, chloride, and bicarbonate, which are found in blood and maintain pH balance in the body

encephalitis — an inflammation/infection of the brain that may cause seizures

endorphins — "feel good" brain chemicals such as dopamine

excitatory neurotransmitters — brain chemicals that increase the electrical discharge of neurons

false positive — a test result in which the patient falsely tests positive due to complicating factors or limitations of the test

fatty acids — the building blocks of dietary lipids

food enzymes — natural chemicals present in all fresh food that contribute to fermentation and chemical breakdown

GABA (Gamma-aminobutyric acid) — an important inhibitory neurotransmitter that prevents calcium from entering the neuron, reducing the electrical action potential

generalized seizures — seizures that involve both halves of the brain

glial cells — cells that provide a support structure in the brain and regulate neurochemicals

glutamate — an excitatory neurotransmitter and amino acid formed from glutamic acid

glutathione peroxidase — an enzyme that protects cell membranes from the damage of free radical molecules

glycine — an important inhibitory neurotransmitter and amino acid

grand mal seizures — seizures that involve body-wide convulsions, now called generalized seizures

hyperglycemia — high levels of blood glucose

hypertrophy — enlargement of tissues or organs from excessive use

hypoglycemia — low levels of blood glucose

hypothyroidism — insufficient thyroid function

hypoxia — a state resulting from insufficient levels of oxygen in the bloodstream

idiopathic epilepsy — epilepsy of an unknown cause

immunoglobulins — a family of antibodies

immunoglobulin A (IgA) — considered to be the body's first line of defense and found in tears, saliva, and mucous membranes

inflammatory bowel syndrome — a general term used to indicate chronic inflammation of the digestive tract

inhibitory neurotransmitters — brain chemicals that decrease neuron discharge

ion channels — molecular "gates" (proteins) within cell membranes that control the flow of ions in and out of a cell

ischemia — an insufficient amount of oxygen delivery to the body's cells

ketogenic diet — a low-carbohydrate, high-fat diet helpful to some human epileptics but which has not been proven especially helpful for dogs

ketones (or **ketone acids**) — a by-product formed during the metabolism of body fat to glucose

kindling — the phenomenon in which seizures become more frequent once a pattern develops

leaky gut syndrome — the condition in which large protein molecules infiltrate the GI tract and initiate an autoimmune response

lipase — an enzyme (produced by the pancreas) responsible for digesting fats (lipids)

lipolysis — the effect cortisol has in breaking down body fat to supply the body with glucose

lymphocytic thyroiditis — an autoimmune disease in which the immune system attacks the thyroid gland; a common cause of hypothyroidism

melatonin — a natural hormone produced in the pineal gland responsible for wake/sleep cycles

meningitis — inflammation/infection of the brain and spinal cord membranes that may cause seizures

metabolism/metabolic — the process by which food is chemically broken down and converted to energy for cell life

MRI (magnetic resonance imaging) — a brain scan that reveals brain structure

neurotransmitters — chemicals that affect neuron activity

pancreatitis — inflammation of the endocrine portion of the pancreas, either chronic or acute in nature

partial seizures — seizures involving only one part of the brain

photosensitive epilepsy — seizures triggered by flickering or flashing lights

polydipsia (PD) — excessive thirst

polyphagia (PP) — excessive hunger

polyuria (PU) — excessive urination

protease — a pancreatic enzyme responsible for digesting dietary proteins

QD — once daily, also abbreviated SID

seizure focus — the area of the brain in which a seizure begins

seizure threshold — the degree of susceptibility to seizures

serum — the fluid portion of the blood

serum biochemical panel — a test that measures liver enzyme function

serum cholesterol and triglyceride concentration test — a test that indicates levels of lipids in the bloodstream

SID — once daily, also abbreviated QD

simple partial seizures — seizures involving only one part of the brain, with no loss or change of consciousness

status epilepticus — continuous or ongoing seizures, potentially life-threatening

sudden aquired retinal degeneration (SARD) — sudden blindness frequently associated with signs of excess cortisol

thyroid hormone — the hormone responsible for regulating the body's metabolic rate

tonic seizures — seizures that cause stiffening of muscles, especially of the back , legs, and neck

tonic-clonic seizures — seizures that cause alternating convulsions and stiffening of muscles, once called grand mal seizures

Type 1 diabetes mellitus — the type of diabetes caused by a destruction of pancreatic beta cells, usually requiring insulin

Bibliography

Animal Protection Institute of America, Sacramento, California, "Pet Food Investigative Report," www.api4animals.org/petfood.htm, May, 1996.

Barry, E., et al, "Ictal Blindness and Status Epilepticus Amauroticus," *Epilepsia*, 26(6): 1985.

Belfield, W.O., "Idiopathic Epilepsy," *Your Animal's Health*, an online newsletter, www.belfield.com, January-February, 1998.

Berti I., et al, "Usefulness of Screening Program for Celiac Disease in Autoimmune Thyroiditis," *Digestive Diseases and Sciences,* 45(2): February, 2000.

Billinghurst, I., *Give Your Dog a Bone: The Practical Commonsense Way to Feed Dogs For a Long Healthy Life*, Australia: self-published, 1993.

Blaylock, R.L., *Excitotoxins: The Taste That Kills*. Santa Fe: Health Press, 1994.

Bourre, J.M., *Brainfood: A Provocative Exploration of the Connection Between What You Eat and How You Think*. Boston: Little, Brown and Company, 1998.

Braund, K.G., (Ed.) "Neurotoxic Disorders," *Clinical Neurology In Small Animals*. New York: International Veterinary Information Service, 2001.

Burkhard, P.R., et al., "Plant-induced Seizures: Reappearance of an Old Problem," *Journal of Neurology*, 246(8): August, 1999.

Carlson, D.G., and Giffin, J.M., *Dog Owner's Home Veterinary Handbook*. New York: Howell Book House, 1992.

Carson, J., "Treating Cluster Seizures with the Rectal and Oral Valium Protocol," www.canine-epilepsy-guardianangels.com, February, 2002.

Claudio, L., et al, "Testing Methods for Developmental Neurotoxicity of Environmental Chemicals," *Toxicology and Applied Pharmacology*, 164(1): April, 2000.

Clemmons, R.M., "Clinical Neurology in a Nutshell," http:// pawcare.com/rclemmons, 2002.

Clemmons, R.M., "Seizure Disorders in Dogs and Cats," http://pawcare.com/rclemmons, January, 2002.

Colorado State University Veterinary Teaching Hospital, "Small Animal Vaccination Protocol," http://www.vth.colostate.edu/vth/savp2.html, February, 2002.

Councell, C., et al, "Coexistence of Celiac and Thyroid Disease," *Gut,* 35(6): June, 1994.

Crook, A., Dawson, S., and Hill, B., "Globoid Cell Leukodystrophy," *Canine Inherited Disease Database*, Atlantic Veterinary College, University of Prince Edward Island, http://www.upei.ca/~cidd/: 2001.

Dakshinamurti, K., et al, "Neuroendocrinology of Pyridoxine Deficiency," *Neuroscience and Biobehavioral Reviews*, 12: 1988.

Dodds, W.J., "Autoimmune Thyroid Disease," *DogWorld,* 77(5): October, 1992.

Dudley, K., "Eliminate Fleas Without Poisons: Integrated Pest Management is a Nontoxic Way to Effectively Control Fleas," *Whole Dog Journal,* 5(3): March, 2002.

Ferran, R., "Gold Bead Implants," *The Pet Tribune*, an online newsletter of the Ludlam-Dixie Animal Clinic, Miami, Florida, http://www.naturalpetdoc.com/pettribune.htm, November-December, 2000.

Field, T., "Massage therapy," *Medical Clinics of North America*, 86(1): January, 2002.

Frankel, P., and Madsen, F., *Stop Homocysteine Through the Methylation Process*. Thousand Oaks, CA: TRC Publications, 1998.

Ganong, W.F., *Review of Medical Physiology*. Norwalk, CT: Appleton & Lange, 1993.

Garcia, M.C., et al, "Effect of Docosahesaenoic Acid on the Synthesis of Phosphatidylserine in Rat Brain Microsomes and c6 Glioma Cells," *Journal of Neurochemistry*, 70(1): January, 1998.

Giroud, M., and Dumas, R., "Epilepsy and Endocrine Modifications," *Encephale*, March-April, 1988.

Gobbi, G., et al, "Celiac Disease, Epilepsy and Cerebral Calcifications," *Lancet*, 340(8817): August, 1992.

Goldstein, M., *The Nature of Animal Healing: The Path to Your Pet's Health, Happiness, and Longevity*. New York: Alfred A Knopf, 1999.

Grabenstein, J.D., *Immuno Facts: Vaccines & Immunologic Drugs*. St. Louis: Facts & Comparisons, 1999.

Haessig, A., et al, "Stress-induced Suppression of the Cellular Immune Reactions: On the Neuroendocrine Control of the Immune System," *Medical Hypotheses*, 46(6): June, 1996.

Horger, B.A., and Roth, R.H., "Stress and Central Amino Acid System," *Neurobiological and Clinical Consequences of Stress: From Adaptation to PTSD*. Lippincott-Raven: Philadelphia, 1995.

Hughes, G.R.V., "The Antiphospholipid Syndrome: Ten Years On," *Lancet*, 342: August, 1993.

Johnstone, C., Knight, D.H., and Lok, J.B., "Epidemiology of Canine Heartworm Disease," http://cal.vet.upenn.edu/parasit/heartworm/hw_3.html, July, 1997.

Kantrowitz, L.B., et al, "Serum Total Thyroxin, Total Triiodothyronine, Free Thyroxin and Thyroxin and Thyrotropin Concentrations in Epileptic Dogs Treated with Anticonvulsants," *Journal of the American Veterinary Medical Association*, 214(12): June, 1999.

Kendall, R.V., *Complementary and Alternative Veterinary Medicine: Principles and Practice*. St. Louis: Mosby, 1997.

Kerr, D.I.B., et al., "Stress and Cortisol Modulation of GABA Receptors," *Stress & Anxiety*, (13): 1990.

Kidd, P.M., *Phosphatydlserine: The Nutrient Building Block that Accelerates all Brain Functions and Counters Alzheimer's*. New Canaan: Keats Publishing, 1998.

Kubler-Ross, E., *On Death and Dying: What the Dying Have to Teach Doctors, Nurses, Clergy, and Their Own Families.* New York: Touchstone Books, 1969.

Kubova, H., Folbergrova, J., and Mares, P., "Seizures Induced by Homocysteine in Rats During Ontogenesis," *Epilepsia*, 36(8): August, 1995.

Lendon, H., and Smith, M.D., *Feed Your Body Right: Understanding Your Individual Body Chemistry for Proper Nutrition Without Guesswork.* New York: Evans and Co. Inc., 1994.

Levin, C.D., *Dogs, Diet and Disease: An Owner's Guide to Diabetes Mellitus, Pancreatitis, Cushing's Disease, and More.* Oregon City: Lantern Publications, 2001.

Lindenbaum, E.S., and Mueller, J.J., "Effects of Pyridoxine on Mice After Immobilization Stress," *Nutrition and Metabolism*, 17: 1974.

Lombard, J., and Germano, C., *The Brain Wellness Plan.* New York: Kensington Publishing Corporation, 1998.

Magaudda, A., et al, "Bilateral Occipital Calcification, Epilepsy and Coeliac Disease: Clinical and Neuroimaging Features of a New Syndrome," *Journal of Neurology, Neurosurgery and Psychiatry*, 56(8): August, 1993.

Mark, J.M., "Seizure Alert Dogs," http://www.vetcentric.com/magazine/magazineArticle.cfm?ARTICLEID=1456, April, 2000.

Martin, A.N., *Foods Pets Die For: Shocking Facts About Pet Food.* Troutdale, OR: New Sage Press, 1997.

Maun, K., "When Your Dog Has Seizures — Coping With a Scary Situation," *Dog Nose News*, 2(3): October, 2001.

Monteleone, P., et al, "Blunting by Chronic Phosphatydlserine Administration of Stress-Induced Activation of the Hypothalamic-Pituitary-Adrenal Axis in Healthy Men," *European Journal of Clinical Pharmacology*, 42(4): 1992.

Mount Sinai Comprehensive Epilepsy Center staff, "Seizure-Provoking Factors," http://epilepsy.med.nyu.edu/Book/provoke.html, October, 2001.

National Institute of Neurological Disorders: "Seizures and Epilepsy," http://www.ninds.nih.gov/health_and_medical/pbs/seizures_and_epilepsy_htr.htm, 2001.

Natori, Y., et al, "Changes of Thyroid Hormone Levels During ACTH Therapy in Epileptic Children," *Rinsho Byori,* (article originally in Japanese) July, 1994.

Northwest Coalition for Alternatives to Pesticides (NCAP) staff, "Managing Fleas Without Poisons," *Journal of Pesticide Reform*, 17(3): Fall, 1997.

Oliver, J.E., Lorenz, M.D., and Kornegay, J.N., *Handbook of Veterinary Neurology, Third Edition*. Philadelphia: WB Saunders Company, 1997.

Olson, L., "Anatomy of a Carnivore and Dietary Needs," *B-Natural's Newsletter,* Spring, 1999.

Osiecki, H., *The Physician's Handbook of Clinical Nutrition*. Kelvin Grove, Australia: Bio Concepts Publishing, 1995.

Panzer, R.B., and Chrisman, C.L., "An Auricular Acupuncture Treatment for Idiopathic Canine Epilepsy: A Preliminary Report," *American Journal of Chinese Medicine*, 22(1): 1994.

Plechner, A.J., and Zucker, M., *Pet Allergies: Remedies for an Epidemic*. Inglewood, CA: Very Healthy Enterprises, 1986.

Podell, M., "The Use of Diazepam per Rectum at Home for the Acute Management of Cluster Seizures in Dogs," *Journal of Veterinary Internal Medicine*, 9(2): 1995.

Raber, J., "Detrimental Effects of Chronic Hypothalamic-Pituitary-Adrenal Axis Activation," *Molecular Neurobiology*, August, 1998.

Richard, A., and Reiter, J., *Epilepsy: A New Approach*. New York: Prentice Hall, 1990.

Rosenberger, B., *Life Itself: Exploring the Realm of the Living Cell*. Oxford: Oxford Press, 1998.

Sapolsky, R.M., *Why Zebras Don't Get Ulcers: An Updated Guide to Stress, Stress Related Disease, and Coping*. New York: W.H. Freeman & Co., 1998.

Sarjeant, D., and Evans, K., *Hard to Swallow: The Truth About Food Additives*. Burnaby, BC: Alive Books, 1999.

Schoen, A.M., "Animal Massage: The Touch That Heals," www.drschoen.com/articles_L2_2_.html, October, 2001.

Schoen, A.M., "Seizures in Dogs & Cats: An Integrative Approach with Natural Options," www.drschoen.com/articles_L2_14_.html, December, 2001.

Schultz, K.R., *The Ultimate Diet: Natural Nutrition for Dogs and Cats*. Decanso, California: Affenbar Ink, 1998.

Scott, D.W., Miller, W.H., and Griffin, C.E., *Muller & Kirk's Small Animal Dermatology*. Philadelphia: W.B. Saunders Co., 2000.

Shames, R., and Shames K.H., *Thyroid Power: Ten Steps to Total Health*. New York: Harper Resource, 2001.

Smith J.B., and Cowchock F.S., "Antiphospholipid Antibodies: Clinical and Laboratory Considerations, Pathophysiology, and Treatment," *Immunology and Allergy Clinics of North America,* 14(4): April, 1994.

Speciale, J., and Stahlbrodt, J.E., "Use of Ocular Compression to Induce Vagal Stimulation and Aid in Controlling Seizures in Seven Dogs," *Journal of the American Veterinary Medical Association*, 214(5): 1999.

Strombeck, D.R., *Home Prepared Dog & Cat Diets: The Healthful Alternative*. Ames: Iowa State University Press, 1999.

Sudha, K., et al, "Oxidative Stress and Antioxidants in Epilepsy," *Clinica Chimica Acta* 303(1-2): January, 2001.

Swift, R., "Milk Thistle: Herbal Wonder," *The Pet Tribune*, an online newsletter, http://www.pettribune.com/1998/040598/9.html, April, 1998.

Tellington-Jones, L., *Getting in TTouch With Your Dog*. N. Promfret, Vermont: Trafalgar Square Publishing, 2001.

Thomas, W.B., "Home Treatment with Rectal Diazepam for Cluster Seizures in Dogs," *Veterinary Clinics of North America: Small Animal Practice*, 30(1): January, 2000.

Tuomisto, L., et al, "Modifying Effects of Histamine on Circadian Rhythms and Neuronal Excitability." *Behavioral Brain Research,* 124(2): October, 2001.

Vliet, E.L., *Screaming to be Heard: Hormone Connections Women Suspect and Doctors Ignore.* New York: M. Evans and Company, Inc., 2001.

Wellington, K., and Jarvis, B., "Silymarin: A Review of its Clinical Properties in the Management of Hepatic Disorders," *BioDrugs*, 15(7): 2001.

Wolfsheimer, K. and Brady, C., "Thyroid Testing in Dogs: A Reference for Dog Breeders and Owners," an article from the Louisiana State University School of Veterinary Medicine, http://www.golden-retriever.com/thyr-lsu.html, November, 2001.

Wulff-Tilford, M.L., and Tilford, G.L., *Herbs for Pets.* Irvine: Bow Tie Press, 1999.

Index

A

ACTH 13, 21, 52
ACTH stimulation test 58
Activated methyl cycle 19
Acupuncture 115
Addison's disease 58, 60
Adenosine triphosphate. *See* ATP
Adrenal gland 13
   Exhaustion 58, 62
Adrenal gland atrophy 46
Adrenocorticotrophic hormone. *See* ACTH
AEDs 75–84, 93, 101
Aggressive behavior 130
Allergic reactions 51, 62
Alpha dog. *See* Pack dynamics: Changes in
Amino acids 16, 50
   Essential (EAAs) 17
   Non-essential (NEAAs) 17
Anemia 62
Animal Protection Institute 46
Antibiotic use 98, 135
Antibodies 50, 60
Antiepileptic drugs. *See* AEDs
Antiphospholipid Antibody Syndrome 60
Apoptosis 148
Appetite. *See* Hunger
Arresting behaviors 125
Arthritis 55
Artificial colors 46
Aspartate 25, 53
ATP 18, 22, 43, 59
Aura 32, 122
Autoimmune disease 49, 59
Autoimmune diseases 60
Autoimmune thyroiditis 143
Axon 22

B

B vitamins 18, 19, 43, 107, 157
   B6/pyridoxine 18
Bach Five Flower Essence 118
BARF. *See* Diet
Belly sling 161

Beta cells 15
BHA 46
BHT 46
Bile 12, 14, 17, 45, 111
Bile acid test 78, 142
Billinghurst, Dr. Ian 97
Bladder stones 55
Blindness 56, 129
   SARD 147
   Training program 148
   Transient Ischemia 147
Blood glucose 15, 16, 52
   Testing 33
Blood sugar. *See* Blood glucose
Blood-brain barrier 21, 53
Bone demineralization 55
Bones 97, 99, 104
Bowel. *See* Intestines
Brain 20
Brainstem 20
Breeding practices 158

C

Calcinosis cutis 55
Calcium 18, 19, 53, 108
   Supplements 95, 100
Carcinogens 46
Cardiac irregularities 53
Catabolism 16, 53
Cedar 156
Celiac disease. *See* Grain intolerance
Cell
   Energy 15
Cell membranes. *See* Membrane
Cerebellum 21
Cerebrospinal fluid 21, 34
Cerebrum 20
Cervical spine 119
Channels. *See* Ion channels
Chemicals 63
Chemistry profile 33
Chiropractic treatment 119
Chloride 18, 25, 79

Cholesterol 53
Circadian rhythms 21, 56
Clemmons, Dr. Roger 107
Clingy behaviors 122
Clonazepam 87
Cluster seizures 75. *See also* Seizures
Cognitive function 56
Collapsed tracheal cartilage 55
Colon. *See* Large intestine
Comfort Measures 159–161
Competitive sports 154–155
Complete blood count (CBC) 33
Complex carbohydrates 48
Computerized Axial Tomography (CAT) Scan 34
Confusion 129
Congestive heart failure 53
Cooling pads 159
Cortisol 13, 16, 47, 66, 111, 127
    Patterns of release 56–57
    Symptoms 52–55
    The High Cortisol Continuum 57, 68
Crates 150, 153
Cruciferous vegetables 145
Cushing's disease 57

D

Dehydration 119
Dendrites 22
Denosyl SD4 109
Dental health 53, 98
DHA 109
Diabetes Mellitus type I 60
Diarrhea 48, 51, 80, 93, 142
Diazepam. *See* Valium
Diet
    BARF. *See* Diet: Raw
Dietary fat 45
Dietary fats. *See* Lipids
Dietary Supplements 107
Diets 37
    Commercial 37–38
        Bioavailability 42
        Chemicals 46
        Fats 45
        Fiber 44
        Grains 48
        High temperatures 40
        Protein sources 40
        Review of 89
        Slowed digestion 44
    Home-cooked 91–97
    Raw / fresh 97–102
    Switching 102–103
Digestive enzymes 95, 103, 111. *See also* Pancreas

Dimethylglycine (DMG 108
Discoid Lupus 60
DMG 108
DNA 59, 63
Docosahexaenoic acid (DHA) 18, 109
Dog food. *See* Diets
Dog training 163. *See also* Seizure alert dogs
Dry Eye Syndrome 148
Durkes Dr. Terry 115
Dyes 46

E

Ear acupuncture points 116
Eggs 92
Ehrlichoisis 30
Electrical charge 22, 25
Electroencephalogram (EEG) 34
Eltroxin 144
Emotional support 163
Encephalitis 30, 64
Endocrine disrupters 63
Endocrine disruptors 47, 61
Enzymes 12, 41–42, 47
    Liver 78
Essential fatty acids 109. *See also* Fatty acids
Essential oils 64
Estrogen 54, 159
Ethoxyquin 46
Excitotoxicity 47
Exercise 119
Eyes. *See* Ophthalmic issues

F

Fatty acids 17, 45, 93
    Essential (EFAs) 17, 43, 45
        Omega 3 17
        Omega 6 17
        Supplements 109
Felbamate 86
Felbatol 86
Firing 25
Flavor enhancers 47, 156
Flea control 156–157
Flight-or-fight 16
Flower essence therapy 118
Focus 31
Food. *See* Diets
Formalin 65
Fragrances 64
Free radicals 18, 63
Frontal lobe 20
Frontal lobe epilepsy 31

G

GABA 18, 19, 44, 56, 64, 81
Gallbladder 12
gamma-aminobutyric acid. *See* GABA
Gamma-Linoleic Acid (GLA) 18, 109
Gastrointestinal (GI) tract 11–12
Genetic expression 19, 59
Genetic tendency 49, 68, 159
Genetics 59
Germs 98
GI upset 80
GLA 109
Glandular extracts 110, 145
Glaucoma 149
Glial cells 21, 46
Glucose 20
Glutamate 25, 48, 53, 95, 104
Glutamic acid 25
Glycogen 16
Goitrogens 94, 145
Gold beads 115
Grain intolerance 48
Grief. *See* Loss

H

Hearing loss 56
Heart disease 53
Heartworm prevention 155–156
Heat intolerance 55, 129
   Comfort measures 159
Hepatic. *See* Liver
Herbs 64, 110, 118
High blood pressure 54
Histamine 51
Home Valium procedure 82
Homocysteine 19, 44, 55
Hunger 62, 106, 129. *See also* Polyphagia
Hydrocephalus 28, 72
Hydrolysis 15
Hypercalcemia 29
Hyperglycemia 52
Hyperparathyroidism 55
Hyperpigmentation 62
Hyperpolarized 25, 79
Hypertension 54
Hypocalcemia 29
Hypoglycemia 29, 48, 93, 119
Hypothalamus 20
Hypothyroidism 61–62
   Diagnosis and treatment 143
   Symptoms 62
Hypoxia 30, 56

I

IBD 51
Ice cream 122
Identification proteins. *See* Proteins: Identification
IgA 50
IgA deficiency 51
IgE 51
IgG 51
IgM 51
Imaging tests 33–34
Immune system 50, 53, 60
Immunoglobulin A 50
Incontinence 53, 138–142
Infections 54, 134–135
   Ear 135
   Kidney 137
   Skin 135
   Urinary Tract (UTIs) 136
Inflammatory bowel disease 51, 60
Insomnia 56
Insulin 15, 53
Intestines 11–12, 50
   Scarring 45
Iodine 61
Ion channels 23
Ions 18, 22, 23
Ischemia 53

J

Jaundice 43

K

Keratoconjunctivitis sicca 60
Ketogenic diet 102
Kidney disease 91, 138
Kidney infection 137–138
Kidneys 12, 30, 79
Kilograms
   Conversion 76
Kindling 64, 75
Kit 121
Klonopin 87

L

L-thyroxine. *See* Thyroid: Hormone
Laboratory tests 33, 80
Lactic acid 48
Large intestine 12
Leaky Gut Syndrome 60
Lecithin 92
Lethargy 62, 78, 80
Levo-thyroxine. *See* Thyroid: Hormone
Lifting dogs 131

Lipids 17
Lipolysis 16, 53
Liver
  Disease 141
  Function 12, 55, 78, 92, 111
Loading dose 77
Loss 1–2
Lupus. *See* Discoid Lupus
Lymphatic system 14, 17, 52
Lymphocytic thyroiditis 61

M

Magnesium 18, 19, 45, 54, 55, 108
  Supplements 95
Magnesium-rich foods 94
Magnetic Resonance Imaging (MRI) 34
Malabsorption 45, 48, 52
Manganese 107
Massage 116
Meat-grinding 100
Medications
  How to hide pills 104
Melatonin 19, 21, 56, 110, 111
Membrane 19, 47, 56, 63, 111. *See also* Cell membrane
Meningitis 30, 34, 64
Mental confusion 56
Mercury (thimerisol) 65
Metabolism
  Normal 14, 145
Methylation 19, 59, 92
Midbrain 20
Milk thistle (Silymarin) 110
Mitochondria 22
Monosodium glutamate. *See* MSG
Mood changes 56
MSG 47, 65, 92, 148
Mucosal barrier 50
Muscle weakness 53, 77, 80
  Comfort measures 160–161
Mysoline 87

N

N-Acetylcystein 108
Neuroendangerment 53
Neuroendocrinology 21
Neuroimmunology 21
Neurons 22
Neurotoxins 63, 65
Neurotransmitters 16, 24, 43
  Excitatory 24, 53
    Aspartate 25
    Glutamate 25
  Inhibitory 24
    GABA 25
    Glycine 25
Notebook 73

O

Oatmeal 93
Occipital lobe 20
Ocular compression 126
Olson, Dr. Lew 44
Omega 3, 6. *See* Fatty acids
Ophthalmic issues 146–149

P

Pacing 56, 76, 86, 129
Pack dynamics
  Changes in 153
Pack issues 151
Pack members
  During seizures 128
Pancreas 11, 42, 52
  Digestive enzymes 12
Pancreatitis 42, 45, 91
Parasite examinations 33
Parasites 54
Parathyroid
  Gland 14
  Hormone 14
Parietal lobe 20
Partial Seizures 31
Pesticides 63, 74
Phenobarbital (Pb) 76–77
Phenols 47, 63, 65
Phosphate 15
Phosphatidyl Serine 111
Phospholipase 47
Phospholipids 18, 22, 43, 47, 56, 60
Phosphorus 18, 55, 108
  Supplements 95
Physical assessment 133
Phytic acid 48
Pine products 64, 156
Pineal gland 21, 56
Pituitary gland 13, 21
Platelet counts 56
Polydipsia 54, 76, 80
Polyphagia 53, 76
Polyuria 54, 76, 80
Portal system 17
Portosystemic shunt 29
Potassium 18, 22, 55
Potassium bromide (KBr) 78–79
Potassium bromide (Pb) 102

Pounds
  Conversion 76
Prednisone 61
Preservatives 46
Primidone 87
Prodromal period 122
Proteins
  Identification 16, 60
Psychological stress 150–155
Puppies 164
  Intestines 45, 51
Pyrethrins 156
Pyrethroids 64
Pyridoxine. *See* B vitamins: B6/pyridoxine

R

Radiograph (x-rays) 34
Rainbow Bridge 164
Ramp 160
Raw meaty bones (RMBs) 99
Receptors 15, 23
Rectal temperature 130
Rectal Valium procedure. *See* Home Valium procedure
Renal. *See* Kidneys
Rescue Remedy 118
Rivotril 87
Rubber mats 161

S

S-adenosylmethionine. *See* SAMe
Salt 61, 79, 80, 102
SAMe 19, 59, 109
SARD 56
Sedation 78, 80
Seizure alert dogs 123–124
Seizure disorders 28–29
Seizure journal 73, 131
Seizure Kit 121
Seizures 57
  Absence 31
  Causes 28–
    30, 42, 44, 46, 47, 53, 54, 56, 62, 63, 64
  Cluster 32
  Focal seizures 31
  Generalized 31
  Grand mal 31
  Partial seizures 31–32
    Complex 32
    Simple 32
  Patterns/cycles 57
  Phases
    Ictal 127
    Postictal 129
    Preictal 122–124

Status epilepticus 32
  What to do 127, 131
Selenium 45, 107
Sensory arrest 125
Separation anxiety 152–153
Serum bile acid concentrations 33
Serum cholinesterase 33
Serum lead levels 33
Serum lipase 42
Shedding 62
Shen Men points 116
Silymarin. *See* Milk thistle (Silymarin)
Sleep 56
Sling 161
Small intestine 11, 12
Sodium 18, 22, 25
Sodium chloride 102
Sodium-potassium pump 26, 54
Soloxine 144
Soy 95, 104
Spinal Tap 34
Startle and shake 125
Status epilepticus **32**, 75, 87. *See also* Seizures
Stomach 11
Storage diseases 29
Stress. *See* Psychological stress. *See* Cortisol
Stress adaptation 57
Strokes 34
Sudden Retinal Degeneration Syndrome. *See* SARD
Supplements 107–109
Surgery 72, 158
Swift, Dr. Russell 110
Synthroid 144

T

Taurine 54
Tellington-Jones, Linda 116
Tellington-Touch 116
Telodendrites 22, 24
Temperature control 20
Temporal lobe 20
Temporal lobe epilepsy 31
Therapeutic level 76, 79
Thermometer 130
Thirst. *See* Polydipsia
Threefold effect 67
Thyroglobulin 61
Thyroid
  Gland 13, 46
  Hormone 13, 54
    T3 13
    T4 13
Thyroid disease. *See* Hypothyroidism
Thyroid stimulating hormone. *See* TSH
Thyroid tests 54, 78, 143

Thyronine. *See* Thyroid: Hormone
Thyroxine hormone. *See* Thyroid: Hormone
Tom cat-style catheter 84
Traveling / trips 154
Treatment philosophies 8
Triglycerides 53
Triiodothyronine. *See* Thyroid: Hormone
TSH 21, 54
Tuarine 108
Tumors 30, 57, 72
Type 1 diabetics 49

U

Urea 43
Urinalysis 33
Urinary incontinence. *See* Incontinence
Urinary Tract Infections (UTIs) 136
Urination 54
Uveitis 56, 149

V

Vaccines 52, 64, 157–158
    Titers 158
Valium 80–83
    Administering rectally 84
    Forms of 81
    Preparing a syringe 83
Vegetable meals 100
Ventriculoperitoneal shunt 72
Veterinary Orthopedic Manipulation 119
Veterinary specialists 7
Vitamin A 18, 19, 45
Vitamin B. *See* B vitamins
Vitamin C 18, 19, 43, 107
Vitamin D 19
Vitamin deficiency 29
Vitamin E 18, 19, 94, 107
Vomiting 80, 142

W

Water consumption 106
Weight 106
Weight conversion 76
Wheat 48
White blood cells 54, 60, 134
Wormers 63, 155

Z

Zinc 45, 107

Notes

Other Books by the Author

"Living With Blind Dogs: A Resource Book and Training Guide for the Owners of Blind and Low-Vision Dogs" by Caroline D. Levin
8.5"x 11" paperback, 182 pages, illustrated, ISBN 0-9672253-0-2
Price: $29.95 plus shipping & handling $5.95 (U.S. & Can.), $15.95 elsewhere

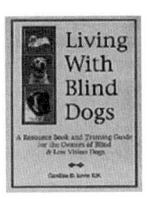

This is the first-ever resource book of its kind. It embodies helpful hints from dozens of blind-dog owners, as well as years of ophthalmic nursing, veterinary, and dog training experiences. Topics include dealing with loss, causes of blindness, how dogs react to blindness, pack interactions, training new skills, toys and games, and more.

"Blind Dogs Stories: Tales of Triumph Humor and Heroism"
by Caroline D. Levin
5.5"x 8.5" paperback, 100 pages, illustrated, ISBN 0-9672253-1-0
Price: $12.95 plus shipping & handling $5.95 (U.S. & Can.), $15.95 elsewhere

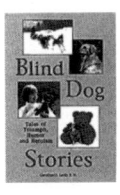

Two dozen short stories, collected from around the world – some of them humorous, some of them heroic, all of them heartwarming. This book demonstrates that blind dogs can live useful and happy lives, offers encouragement to blind-dog owners, and celebrates the beauty of the human-canine bond.

"Dogs, Diet, and Disease: An Owner's Guide to Diabetes Mellitus, Pancreatitis, Cushing's Disease, and More" by Caroline D. Levin
8.5"x 11" paperback, 180 pages, illustrated, ISBN 0-9672253-2-9
Price: $29.95 plus shipping & handling $5.95 (U.S. & Can.), $15.95 elsewhere

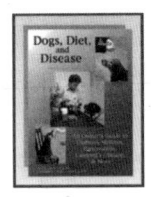

Maxwell Award Winner: *Best Healthcare Book 2001*! Provides indepth instructions to help owners care for chronically ill dogs. Discusses numerous metabolic/digestive/endocrine and immune system processes, diet, nutrition, insulin injections. Cushing's (and SARD) treatments, liver kidney, bladder issues & more.

Ordering:
Shipment is by Priority Mail: 1-3 day delivery in the U.S. For credit card orders, please phone, fax, or visit our website. Make checks payable, (in U. S. funds, on U.S. banks, please) and mail to:

Lantern Publications phone and fax: **(503) 631-3491**
18709 S. Grasle Road email: publisher@petcarebooks.com
Oregon City, OR 97045-8899 USA website: http://www.petcarebooks.com